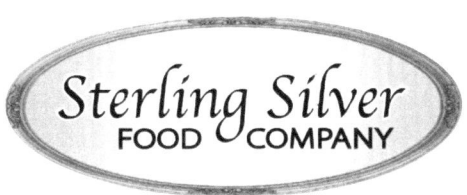

Gluten Free Guide

and

Cook Book

Contact: sterlingsilverfood@gmail.com
Copyright © 2014 by Nancy Shulenberger
First Edition 2014

For My Beloved Shuly

Acknowledgements

From Philadelphia pepper pot soup to chocolate fudge Easter eggs, from pigs' feet souse to live Dungeness crab, my Dad taught me how to cook. He also taught me to love good food and explore fearlessly the flavors of the world. This business and this cookbook really began fifty years ago at my father's side. A few of the recipes in this book are his (minus the pigs' feet souse – although if you email me at sterlingsilverfood@gmail.com, I'll send it to you!).

Mom – beautiful, classy, and wonderfully funny – encouraged me to venture forth in the kitchen and never complained when she had to follow behind to re-clean the less than pristine bowls and cabinet knobs. She loved to entertain in the era of fancy dinner parties, and set the most beautiful table. Her flower arrangements were spectacular, framed by freshly pressed damask linens and her sterling silver flatware. The Sterling Silver Food Company name is a nod to my mother's elegant generosity. Mom and Dad, I miss you every day.

My commercial kitchen family, Heidi, Bob, Rob, Barbara, and Bryce have all provided so much guidance and even loaned me a dozen eggs on occasion. More importantly, they continue to offer information on the local food industry goings-on as well as regular and consistent laughs. The book's front and back covers were lovingly created by the always brilliant Joan Selix Berman.

My delightful daughters Katie and Allison have supported and encouraged me throughout this process. And heck! Without their Celiac Disease, we'd still be living in Wheat Land!

Finally, my husband Chris (aka Shuly) has been behind me 100% during these challenging years. He never complained about my crazy schedule or lack of revenue. Thank you, my dear, for our years together and your unwavering love and support.

Table of Contents

		Introduction	1
One		What's It All About, GF?	3
Two		Don't Eat This – Reading Labels	7
Three		Crumbs, Crumbs Everywhere – Contamination	12
Four		On Beyond Broccoli – Nutrition	16
Five		The Great Unknown - Dining Out	18
Six		GF and Kids	21
Seven		Travel – Senza Glutine in Italia	25
Eight		Cooking 101 – Basic GF Concepts	29
		Recipes – Oh Good, Now We Get To Cook!	
	1.	Life is Short – Lets's Make Dessert First	37
	2.	Loaves	58
	3.	Soups	67
	4.	Salads	73
	5.	Main Courses	83
	6.	Side Dishes	93
	7.	Confections	99
	8.	Granola – The Beginning and the End	105
Recipe Index			107

Introduction

Welcome to the Sterling Silver Food Company, where everything we make is deliciously gluten free. If you are new to the gluten free experience, fear not, and read on. The path before you is brighter now than ever before. With the explosive growth of the diagnosis of Celiac Disease (and gluten intolerance) in the United States, gluten free foods have become very much in demand and decidedly more easily available. The National Institutes of Health estimates that over 3 million Americans (nearly1% of the population) suffer from Celiac Disease. When gluten intolerant individuals are included, the number increases dramatically. Serbian tennis star, Novak Djokovik, who was diagnosed with a gluten intolerance in 2010, switched to a gluten free diet and since that time, he has become the first player to win the Australian Open three years in a row. National food companies have created gluten free versions of their most popular products and they don't seem to be slowing down. For the home cook, creating delicious gluten free dishes can be daunting at first, but with a full understanding of ingredients and methods, and some creative and flavorful recipes, it can be a wonderful step forward.

Our gluten free journey began in 2005 when my younger daughter Allison contracted a nasty stomach flu and had difficulty recovering. As a conscientious mother, I kept giving her traditional tummy food – chicken noodle soup and saltine crackers! Three months later, she had transformed from a slender, athletic 6th grader to a gaunt, colorless wraith. She had lost a good deal of weight and, at an age when

1

young people are customarily growing like weeds, she leveled off. She had always been taller than her older sister at the same age (growing has been a competitive sport in our household for many years), but she lost serious ground during this challenging time. Her doctor was unsure of the diagnosis and he tried a number of dietary changes, none of which was successful. Fortunately (and unfortunately), at this point in our story, two members of our extended family were diagnosed with Celiac Disease. With the understanding that Celiac has a genetic component (thank you, husband dear), we asked the doctor to run some celiac identifying blood tests. The results were not 100% conclusive, but a window had been opened. A follow-up endoscopy and biopsy confirmed the diagnosis. Shortly thereafter, big sister Katie developed Celiac Disease as well. We were now embarking on an entirely new eating plan – Gluten Free.

After relocating to the beautiful Rogue Valley of Southern Oregon in 2009, it seemed imperative that the new insights and recipes developed with love for my children should be shared, and Sterling Silver Food Company was born. If you are new to the gluten free community or are looking for a refresher and some inspiration, I will offer tips and insights about reading labels, nutrition, contamination, dining out, children's issues, which will be followed by a collection of community tested and approved recipes.

The world is changing in our favor. Eating a gluten free diet is not as difficult as it used to be. Armed with this information and your own creative spirit, you will find joy in the kitchen again.

Oh, and Allison? She started growing again. Now, at age 20, she is 6 feet tall. Yes, taller than Katie. It's nothing a little quinoa can't cure!

One

What's it all about - GF

So what can you eat on a gluten free diet? Other than Fritos and fruit? No wheat, rye, or barley. OK. But how can you determine the gluten status of a bottle or box? Crispix cereal says it has rice on one side and corn on the other - no problem. Except for the barley malt flavoring in the cereal which is also found in *corn* flakes and *rice* krispies. How about that green taco sauce that used to be in the Fiesta cabbage slaw recipe? Bad choice - modified food starch. (I had to toss an entire large head of shredded cabbage for that mistake.) Oh, and soy sauce? That has wheat. So when we went to our favorite Chinese restaurant, we just asked them to leave out the soy sauce from our dishes. Wrong again. Most Chinese restaurants don't wash their woks after every dish. They might not include the soy in your Szechuan chicken, but there is residual from the broccoli beef that was prepared previously.

What is gluten? And what is Celiac Disease?

Gluten is a complex of two protein molecules, one a very long chain, which is found in wheat, rye, and barley. Oats have a different

3

form of gluten which has shown to be problematic for some extremely reactive Celiacs. Because oats and wheat/rye/barley are frequently grown and processed in common locations, there is a very high incidence of contamination of the oats which is what makes them inedible for individuals on a strict GF diet. Gluten free oats are available on the market, however. Glutinous rice is a different thing altogether and not an issue in a gluten free diet. Gluten provides the stretch and the structure for breads and other baked goods. It also is used quite extensively for texture and thickness in sauces. The problem with gluten is that some people's bodies have developed a reaction to the ingestion of gluten. Introducing Celiac Disease.

Celiac Disease is an autoimmune condition which causes the body to attack the gluten molecule when it arrives in the intestines. Unfortunately, when the body attacks the gluten, it inadvertently attacks the villi in the lining of the small intestines at the same time, partly destroying them. The villi are the pathways into the blood stream. If they are damaged, then it is difficult to absorb certain nutrients. Many long-term undiagnosed celiacs have problems with anemia because they cannot get enough iron from their diets – often necessitating an iron supplement. Calcium absorption can be impacted as well, which may lead to osteoporosis. Although dairy products have no relationship to gluten, the lactase enzyme that is required to metabolize the lactose found in milk is located on the tip of the villi so that many celiac sufferers exhibit the symptoms of lactose intolerance. Once their intestines have healed, milk products might no longer cause problems.

Fortunately, the "cure" for Celiac Disease is simple and difficult at the same time - a 100% gluten free diet. Without the constant

4

introduction of gluten into the intestines, the autoimmune response is not triggered and the attacks on the villi cease. The villi are then able to heal and the absorption of nutrients resumes.

The symptoms of Celiac Disease are multiple and varied, which is why it is often difficult to diagnose. Intestinal difficulties, including bloating, abdominal pain, and diarrhea are frequent, but so are increased migraines, menstruation problems, joint pain, muscle cramps, mouth sores, anemia, and the inability to maintain a healthy weight (weight loss). The skin condition dermatitis herpetiformis, an itchy, blistering disease which usually appears on the torso, scalp, and buttocks is also associated with the ingestion of gluten. Unfortunately, some patients are asymptomatic and even though there is internal damage, they don't feel sick and therefore have more of a challenge adhering to a gluten free diet. As the awareness of gluten as a prominent food allergen grows, so does the availability of gluten free foods. Physicians are also more aware of the prevalence of Celiac Disease in the population, and the time between the onset of symptoms and a conclusive diagnosis is shorter. In the past, many people suffered for years without knowing what caused their difficulties.

Testing for Celiac Disease has improved as well. Initially, blood tests can determine the existence of certain antibodies which indicate that the immune system is working against the ingestion of gluten. However, if you suspect that you might have Celiac Disease, it is important that you be tested prior to beginning a gluten free eating regimen. As soon as you eliminate gluten from your diet, your body begins to heal and the antibodies will no longer be present. You will test negative for Celiac Disease. If you wish to be tested for a confirmed diagnosis after changing your diet to gluten free, you will have to resume ingestion of gluten for 6-8 weeks or more in order to develop the antibodies. This means you will have to make yourself sick again! The other more invasive but more conclusive test, involves an endoscopy and biopsy of the tissues of the small intestine. A camera pill may also be used to take photographs of the intestines which will be recorded for your doctor's review. These tests will also produce a negative result if the patient has been on a gluten free diet for enough time to regenerate the villi.

There is also genetic testing of DNA which can be performed from a cheek swab. This will identify the genes linked to celiac disease and to gluten sensitivity. In other words, it looks not only at the sensitivity to gliaden (one of the gluten proteins found in wheat), but to others as well.

Whether or not it is a factor in the increase in celiac diagnoses, wheat seems to be an ingredient in a much larger percentage of the food that we consume than in the past. As our lives become busier and we balance careers and families, the multi-billion dollar fast food and processed food industries have stepped in to offer their own solutions. They have provided us with quick and easy meals – complete with extensive ingredients lists containing many items that would probably be better left inside the box and not in our bodies. Real food doesn't require an ingredients list. Fresh fruits, vegetables, and unprocessed meats are always good for us and are always gluten free.

Two

Don't Eat This – Reading Labels

At first, the prospect of embarking on a gluten free diet seems daunting. "I can't eat anything!" When you evaluate your current eating habits, it will seem impossible. It's not. But you will need to learn about the specific items/grains that are forbidden and how to identify them. Knowing that you must avoid wheat, rye, and barley means that you should be able to spot the different forms of the evil grains. They include:

- Bulgur
- Durum
- Farina
- Semolina
- Spelt (which is often touted as a wheat alternative, but it is still GF forbidden)
- Einkorn Wheat
- Graham Flour
- Couscous (which isn't a separate grain, but a tiny form of pasta)

- Rye
- Triticale (a wheat/rye hybrid)
- Barley
- Barley Malt

Perhaps more helpful than this group, is a list of the grains that are going to become your new best friends:

- Arrowroot
- Amaranth
- Quinoa
- Buckwheat
- Corn
- Rice, Brown Rice
- Tapioca
- Gluten Free Flours (including soy, potato, bean, rice, corn)
- Millet

Let's face it, these days most of us who are armed with a grocery list don't have the luxury of time to dawdle over the ingredients itemized on everything we buy. We're commuting, working multiple jobs, managing our children's busy lives, trying to keep fit, and hoping to put a reasonable meal on the table at night.

If you have elected to follow a gluten free diet, either by choice or by medical necessity, you have entered a no-man's land. Initially, you will need to read labels. In the Food and Drug Administration's report "Approaches to Establish Thresholds for Major Food Allergens and for Gluten in Food" – March 2006, eight major food allergens were identified which account for 90% of all allergic reactions. They are milk, eggs, fish, crustacean shellfish, tree nuts, peanuts, wheat, and soybeans.

Proper food labeling requires that these items be clearly identified. Be careful with labeling by smaller producers. There are several baking companies in Southern Oregon whose ingredient lists are just plain wrong, as well as other outfits that bake both gluten-full and gluten free products in the same facility without proper notification. Obviously, an item that specifies that it contains wheat is not gluten free, but what about rye and barley? They are not on the FDA list, so you must look for them. Again, fresh fruits, vegetables, legumes, and unprocessed meats are all gluten free. Let's load up on those! Not only do they eliminate the reading-labels problem, but they provide the best nutrition.

On the other end of the spectrum are the foods with an ingredients list so long and filled with so many poly-syllabic words, that you don't really know what you're eating. Let's just cross these off entirely. After some practice, you will become quite adept at scanning an ingredients list for problematic items.

In the middle of these two ends, reside the semi-processed foods that will satisfy your family, and make your life a little bit easier. After a long work day, choosing Alexia's Waffle Fries (frozen) over my recipe for roasted potatoes (pg. 93) and serving them hot from the oven with a green salad and a Costco rotisserie chicken is just fine every now and again. (The Costco chicken label used to include modified food starch, but they clarified the issue by indicating that it is modified corn starch. Costco, as a retailer, is very aware of gluten sensitivity and they carry many self-identified Gluten Free products.) Modified Food Starch, unless it is specified as corn, potato, tapioca etc., should not be consumed. Malt or malt flavoring comes from barley – which means no regular beer, no Ovaltine, and no Whoppers candies.

As you discover these gluten free items that fit into your culinary plan, make a note of them. But if packaging changes, or it becomes "new and improved", then be sure to read the label again. "Original" Rice-a-Roni with wild rice used to be gluten free, but they changed the formula and we can no longer eat it.

So many more manufacturers are getting on the band wagon now. Eight years ago, we had to scour the bottom shelves at the rear of the health food store across town to find odd-tasting, funny-textured gluten free products. Now, nearly every grocery store, mega or local, has a dedicated gluten free section, with many additional delicious offerings throughout the store. There are gluten free Chex cereals, gluten free Bisquik, and gluten free Betty Crocker cake mixes, as well as a myriad of new manufacturers. Kinnickinnick (we love their pancake mix!), Pamela's, and Tom Sawyer's Gluten Free Flour (glutenfreeflour.com) are just a few.

As far as snacking goes, while plain tortilla or potato chips are safe choices, some of the flavored chips don't work for GF. Read the labels. Start at the bottom of the ingredients list where it says "contains" or "allergens". If it says "wheat", your decision is made for you. If not, you still need to read the whole label. The best chip choices say "potatoes, oil, salt", or "corn, oil, lime, salt".

Watch out for salad dressings, chicken or beef broth, some condiments, and even things like bacon or ham that have been cured with soy sauce. Really. Some medicines use wheat as a texturizing/binding ingredient Also notify your pharmacist of your issues with gluten, and be certain to notify a hospital as well if you happen to be checking in. If you are severely reactive, you might consider wearing a Medic Alert bracelet.

Ultimately, if you're not sure after reading the label, and it's a product that you would like to purchase, either investigate the manufacturer's website's nutritional information and allergen listings, or call the manufacturer directly. By doing this simple thing, we learned that See's Candies are gluten free, as are Mike'n Ikes (even though the label lists modified food starch – it's corn). On the other hand, when we called the manufacturer of one particular antacid product, the customer service agent did not know if their medicine was gluten free or not!

Even though simple logic tells you that a certain food item just can't contain gluten, you might possibly be wrong. And, depending on the severity of your allergic reaction, do you really want to take that chance? Read labels. Green taco sauce? It has gluten in it.

Three

Crumbs Crumbs Everywhere - Contamination

When our older daughter was newly diagnosed, she joined a friend for lunch at a local restaurant that is known for its sandwiches, soups, and salads. She approached the young woman at the counter with her ingredient questions and spent a good fifteen minutes explaining gluten and why she could not eat a sandwich. They considered various options and, after a trip into the kitchen to read marinade ingredients, the server found a grilled chicken salad that was gluten free. The extra effort was much appreciated, and my daughter sat down and awaited her salad. When it arrived, it looked delicious. But after all of that discussion about gluten and wheat, the server had topped the gluten free chicken salad with a nice big slice of their signature sourdough bread. Now, here comes the difficult part. Katie had to explain that she couldn't eat the bread, but more importantly, she couldn't eat the salad underneath the bread, even if it was removed. A whole new salad had to be made. Hopefully, that server wasn't charged for the mistake.

Gluten is a molecule, remember? That means that it's very small, right? So if you have a piece of sliced bread on your chicken salad, then it's likely that a crumb of that bread might have landed on the lettuce of that salad. The crumb of bread contains many gluten molecules, which means that if you eat that contaminated salad, you will consume gluten. The cilia in your intestines don't care how many molecules of gluten you eat. They don't like any of them.

Contamination is a significant issue, even in a very conscientious household. If you dip your knife into the mustard for your pastrami sandwich on rye, fine. If you dip it twice, that's not so fine. You have just transferred gluten from your slice of bread into the mustard jar for the rest of the family to enjoy. There are several ways to avoid this problem. Many condiments are available in squeeze bottles, which eliminates the double-dipping knife problem, but they are expensive and contain too small a volume for a busy household. Having duplicate containers of mustard, mayonnaise, butter, and jam with clear GF identifiers on the top is another possibility, although that can create a very crowded refrigerator (color coded stickers also can be used to make a clear identification of the GF items). In our household, we have a combined solution. For some items we have separate GF and non-GF containers, and for others, we are on the honor system. There is no double-dipping in the mustard, and if you do, you fess up immediately and mark the lid of the jar with NON GF in big bold letters - which also necessitates writing mustard on the grocery list, with lots of mea culpas and groveling. It seems to work. Jam is only consumed by half of our family – one on the GF side and one on the wheat-a-saurus side. Therefore, we have developed a habit of serving some jam onto a dish

13

with a spoon before spreading it onto toast. Some combination of these ideas will probably work in your family if you continue to provide traditional breads for your non-Celiac members. You might also decide that it's not worth the hassle and make your entire house 100% gluten free. That solves the problem completely.

Aside from errant knives in mustard, a significant issue with contamination deals with ingredients that can become airborne. Flour. Wheat flour. If you bake at all, then your kitchen has little flour molecules all over the place. Your stand mixer, electric mixer, bread maker, and food processor are all contaminated. If you make homemade wheat bread and you slice it on the wooden cutting board, you have even more contamination. We elected to banish all non-GF baking (and cooking) ingredients from our kitchen, which required us to become really good at GF baking so that nobody ever complained about the food production in our house.

Finding a good replacement for wheat flour was a huge part of this decision, and we found one that we like very much. In fact, Tom Sawyer's Gluten Free Flour (which can be found at www.glutenfreeflour.com) is the one that is used almost exclusively in the Sterling Silver Food Company kitchen. They have two different formulas. One has unflavored gelatin in it – not vegetarian, and the other does not and can be used in vegetarian/vegan cooking.

It really is not that difficult to prepare gluten free meals, and if they are well made and flavorful, it makes a lot of sense that everyone in your household will eat and enjoy them. Don't make two pots of pasta, when the Tinkyada brand GF pasta is delicious. There is not one thing that is cooked in our house that has gluten in it. The only non – GF

14

items that cross our threshold in a grocery bag are bread products and they are stored separately. We have two toasters that are kept in different cupboards. All other condiments and cooking products are gluten free. Even though our daughters are away at college now, we haven't changed our ways. We'd like it if they would come back and visit now and again (and not just to do laundry), so the kitchen remains GF friendly.

If you make a grilled cheese sandwich in the fry pan with wheat bread, that's fine as long as you wash the pan thoroughly. At the beginning of your gluten free odyssey, you do not need to buy all new cooking equipment (except maybe for the toaster, which is almost impossible to decontaminate completely). A very thorough cleaning will remove any lingering gluten.

Four

On Beyond Broccoli - Nutrition

Good nutrition and good health come from a well-balanced diet which includes lots of fresh fruits and vegetables, grains, and proteins. Vitamins, minerals, and fiber are essential to good nutrition as well, and many of these come from grains. Whole wheat is a high fiber grain which contains iron, magnesium, phosphorus, potassium, zinc, manganese, selenium, calcium, protein, and vitamin B6. It can be a powerful part of a good diet. Although many of these nutrients can be found in the meat, grain, and vegetable realm, replacing wheat isn't always easy.

The first alternatives that come to mind for a newly diagnosed celiac, it seems, are rice, corn, and potatoes. But none of these three come anywhere close to the nutritional value found in wheat, so gluten free consumers must look to other sources for replacements. Enter the ancient grains. Quinoa, millet, and amaranth are making a come-back in the kitchen. They are lovely additions to soups, breads, and cereals. Whole quinoa is a delightful swap for the bulgur wheat in tabouleh salad (recipe found on page 79), and quinoa flakes are found in my granola

16

(page 105). Buckwheat is not related to wheat and is a wonderful grain for hot cereal or buckwheat flour for pancakes.

Some options for nutritional alternatives for wheat are:

- Iron – green leafy vegetables, beef, potatoes, tomatoes
- Magnesium – chives, basil, sage, pumpkin seeds, sesame seeds, peanuts
- Phosphorous – milk, baking powder, rice, GF oats, amaranth, salmon, cod
- Potassium – apricots, bananas, parsley, celery, bell peppers, quinoa, amaranth, oats
- Zinc – oysters, wild rice, mushrooms, beef
- Manganese – grape leaves, bell peppers, GF oats, garlic, brown rice, millet, amaranth, quinoa
- Selenium – turkey, brazil nuts,
- Calcium – corn meal, amaranth, milk, cheese, sesame seeds, chia seeds, almonds
- Protein – meat, legumes, eggs, cheese, seaweed, fish
- Vitamin B6 – amaranth, brown rice flour, corn, leeks, potatoes, shallots, onions
- Fiber – buckwheat, pumpkin, quinoa, sun dried tomatoes, lentils and other beans

This list is obviously not exhaustive by any means. It is merely an example of the kinds of food decisions that you will be making now that wheat is no longer on the menu. There are many ways to ensure that your body stays healthy, particularly through your healing phase.

Five

The Great Beyond – Dining Out

Once you have mastered your own kitchen environment, it's time to venture out into restaurant-land. Although it has become dramatically easier recently, you still need to become a very good investigator.

Early on in our gluten free adventure, my daughter's soccer team had an end of season dinner at a local pizza and pasta restaurant. The day before the event, I checked their menu and found that, other than lettuce, there was nothing she could eat. So I spoke to the manager, asking if he would cook a piece of meat for her that we provided. He said yes with a smile, pulled out a clean pan and brought her a nice meal. She was able to join in the group activity without feeling like an outsider. And truth be told, the other kids at the table were eyeing her dinner with some interest.

Many chain restaurants have separate gluten free menus. PF Chang's, Legal Seafood in Boston, The Cheesecake Factory, UNO Pizzeria and Grill, and Outback Steakhouse are just a few of the spots that have seen the light. Be cautious with sandwich chains that have assembly line situations. I have personally seen regular bread crumbs brushed into the lettuce bin. Fine dining establishments are generally very happy to prepare a special gluten free meal, or at least indicate which menu items are safe to eat. While enjoying dinner at Farallon in San Francisco not too long ago (an incredibly special treat), my daughter explained her gluten free status to the server. He replaced the customary plate of bread at the beginning of our meal with some delectable fried potatoes. He told us exactly which dishes were the best options, and made certain that her meal was not only spectacularly delicious, but safe to eat as well.

If your young children are Celiac, then teach them how to ask the right questions about ingredients, marinades (soy sauce in some Mexican restaurants), and cooking/grilling environments. The more they learn about dining out, and the more they take responsibility for their eating, the better consumers they will be. You will also be able to relax when they go out with other families when you are not present. Most servers – at least, those interested in earning a nice tip – when asked politely, are more than willing to be helpful. And they often don't mind if you ask for special treatment – cooking your chicken in a clean pan instead of on the contaminated grill, for example. If that is not the case, you might speak to the manager or consider eating elsewhere. Some restaurants serve so many dishes that have gluten in them that the environment is really not conducive to your having a safe and enjoyable meal. Just don't eat there. Although omelets are usually a good breakfast choice, IHOP pancake restaurants mix pancake batter into the eggs. On the other side of the coin, In-n-Out Burger, a place that has always been very accommodating to requests for "protein-style" (wrapped in lettuce) burgers which are cooked separately from the regular burgers, now has an "allergy" button on their registers which notifies the cooking staff without complicated explanations. Their fries are made from freshly cut potatoes and are also safe, unlike those at most fast food restaurants, which are made from a mashed and reconstituted potato product that is rarely gluten free.

If a restaurant has a deep fryer, be sure to ask if they cook the chimichangas (a fried flour tortilla burrito) in the same oil as the chips. If they cook the fried chicken in the same oil that they fry their potatoes, make a different choice.

If you have a favorite pre-Celiac Italian restaurant, where you are a well-known and frequent diner, then consider bringing a bag of gluten free pasta with you and asking them to boil a clean pot of water for your meal (double checking their sauces, of course). It's certainly been done. And again, if that small restaurant realizes that doing you a favor like that will mean a more consistent customer for them, it's certainly a win-win situation.

As we gluten free folk take over the world, more and more restaurants are trying to capture our business and our devotion by allowing us to relax with a meal, knowing that we won't regret it in the morning. It's so smart.

Six

GF and Kids

Some children are born with full blown Celiac Disease, and some (like my two daughters) develop it later in their young lives. Each stage has its challenges. Very young children may have difficulty communicating their symptoms, although their discomfort is usually readily apparent! Some newborns may have problems with formulas, or even with breast milk if the mother is consuming gluten. Although there is no medical proof, anecdotal evidence from mothers who have changed to a gluten free eating program indicates that babies previously labeled "colicky" might actually have Celiac Disease.

The world has become a more welcoming place for those wishing to eat gluten free, but the life of a child can still be difficult with the removal of all gluten. What about his best friend's birthday party complete with goldfish crackers and chocolate cake? Or her end-of-season soccer party held at a pizza parlor. What is to be done with sleep overs? As a parent, you cannot chase him around town with a bag of Glutino pretzels and a package of Van's gluten free frozen waffles.

Teaching your child about her condition is vital so that she eventually will be able to take full responsibility for her food intake.

21

Teaching others isn't always easy, however. For every parent like Pam or Theresa, who went out of their way to provide wonderful gluten free meals when Allison went over to visit their homes, there were others who thought giving Katie an apple with a flag stuck in the top was equivalent to a custom home made individual cake for every other member of the team. You can do your part to help to educate others ("Trader Joe's sells a wonderful gluten free brownie mix that is delicious for everyone!") to avoid some of these hurtful circumstances.

Day care providers should be fully apprised of your child's food needs. If it is a facility that offers meals and snacks, you will need to educate the owner or, if you don't feel comfortable, you should provide the food yourself. Although it definitely doesn't count in the snack category, Play Doh has wheat in it. Katie absolutely remembers tasting it in pre-school. Depending on your child's sensitivity, even playing with it could be hazardous. Little hands go into little mouths.

In school, providing a brown bag lunch is probably the best option. A busy school cafeteria is not likely to offer very many alternatives that will keep your child safe. Salad bars can be very dangerous. Even adult salad bars can be a hazard. The crouton spoon might be used to serve up carrots and now you have contamination. You should certainly speak to your child's teacher at the beginning of the school year to alert him to the situation. If children are permitted to bring treats on their birthdays for the whole class, you might ask the teacher to let you know that this is happening so that you can provide something for your child. The one thing that Allison has mentioned about her journey through middle and high school, is that she often felt left out, and sometimes felt slighted. One after-season team party was held at Freddy's Pizza and she had a plain baked potato for dinner.

Her trip to Washington D.C. in eighth grade was completely different. The teachers on the trip made an extra effort to provide GF meals. They would even pick up a take-out meal for her at a steak place on the way to the pasta restaurant where the rest of the group was eating. Summer camp sounds like a potential nightmare, and it can be. But Mountain Meadow Ranch in Susanville, California made it all so easy. Prior to the girls' arrival, the owner of the camp reviewed the nightly menus with me over the phone, and determined how many meals were NOT gluten free. Then I prepared and froze some individual portions of food for them to take, augmented with a few store-bought frozen meals. We delivered them all to the camp freezer, along with loaves of GF bread, cookies, and condiments (for sandwiches) when we arrived and the girls had two weeks of easy food and a fantastic experience.

There are little things that can be tricky. The girls can't always try new foods because they are not able to identify something without a label. They can't share food with their friends, or even sodas because the can or straw might be contaminated.

Going off to college presents another set of issues. Every school is different and some are better than others at providing good, nutritious, edible, and gluten free food. Our cousin was assigned to a nutritionist when she went to college, and soon realized that she was in trouble when the woman told her she could eat the salad that was being offered one evening – only to discover that it was *macaroni* salad! She ended up cooking her own meals in a little dorm kitchen, which wasn't exactly ideal, but it allowed her to eat decently and safely during her college years. Pizza and beer parties were definitely out of the question, and I am sure that she felt like "the other" when those events came up.

Being a college athlete adds another level of challenge. The assistant coach who was responsible for feeding Katie's basketball team after an away game selected pasta, garlic bread, and Caesar salad for the other players – and a bag of lettuce for her! Remember that <u>you</u> initially thought eating a gluten free diet was going to be impossible, so try to understand that others attempting to serve a celiac individual might feel completely out to sea as well. We can try to be patient – although the protective Mother Bear may appear at any moment!

Um. Kissing. Maybe the only word that needs to be added to this explanation is – contamination. If your boyfriend just ate regular pizza, and you have Celiac Disease, you shouldn't kiss him. There.

There is ongoing research being pursued for earlier, simpler, and more definitive testing for Celiac Disease. Gluten free foods are available almost everywhere now, and restaurants are realizing that accommodating their GF guests is good for business. Children can grow and thrive with a little guidance and encouragement from you.

Seven

Travel – Senza Glutine in Italia

Quickly – a word association quiz.

ITALY.......... _____

Maybe you said Rome. Maybe you said The Sistine Chapel, The Catacombs, or Tuscany. If you are a foodie, you might have said pasta, pizza, or bread. So if you have visions of seeing the Coliseum at night, or the magnificent art in the Vatican museum, you will probably just have to bring your own food. Or starve. No pasta Bolognese for you! Well, maybe there might be something to eat in Rome, but in Siena, Lucca, Positano, or near Pompeii? The Isle of Capri? Never happen, right? Wrong. Italy and most of Europe are far ahead of the United States in understanding and providing gluten free fabulousness. The whole world is coming over to our side.

We spent three weeks in Italy in 2013. We had one week in Rome, one week in the Tuscan hills outside of Florence, and one week in Positano (on the Amalfi Coast). We did not starve. It was the trip of a

25

lifetime – with the food of a lifetime to go with it. The two most important words we learned before we left were "senza glutine". If you wish to travel to other countries, here you go:

France – sans gluten

Spain – sin gluten

Germany – glutenfrei

Sweden – glutenfri

Hungary – glutenmentes

The Netherlands – glutenvrij

Greece - χωρίς γλουτένη

There was even a restaurant directly across the street from the Duomo in Florence that had a sign out front advertising that they had a large gluten free menu and could accommodate celiacs. The pizza and hot rolls were so good there, we went back a second time. Not every restaurant had gluten free pizza, but most of them had pasta, or the servers could identify the meats, vegetables, and other items on the menu that we could eat. The simple foods were most consistently safe and lovely. Caprese salad is always a good choice. And every bowl of minestrone soup we enjoyed did not have pasta in it. Wonderful! Our Italian language mastery was marginal at best, but with those two little magic words, meals were so enjoyable and worry free.

Because there were four of us traveling together, and because we were spending a week in each of the three locations, we rented apartments (and a house outside of Florence) instead of staying in hotels. The lodging cost for four adults was more affordable for a whole house than for two hotel rooms or a suite. The girls don't share a room with us anymore. We snore. One of the best parts of having a home was being able to cook some of our own meals. Restaurant food in Italy is pricy, so we often ate lunch out, and dinner at home. Shopping in the local markets was a real treat. In Rome, our apartment was on the Via de Coronari (close to the Piazza Navona) and there was a wonderful little grocery store across the street. They had plenty of GF items – pasta, bread, crackers, and cookies. Buying fresh cheeses, sliced meats, and olives (Oh! The olives!) from our local store made us feel more like locals. Well-fed locals.

The most exciting discovery of the trip was made in Florence. We were staying in a charming little house up in the hills, nestled between olive groves and vineyards. Our host explained to us that in order to drive in Florence, you needed to have a special (and expensive) permit for the car. We did not have this permit. Nor were we very keen to brave the narrow streets of the city. It was much better to drive to the local bus stop, park the car and ride into town. On the way through the traffic and across the Arno River, I suggested to Allison that she Google search Firenze pasticceria (pastry shop) senza glutine. Up popped the name of a store across town from our intended destination. What better excuse for a long walk on the beautiful streets of Florence than the enticement of pastries at the end? It was a long walk. Through the business district. Not where we expected to go. It rained a little. We were getting impatient and frustrated. What's the word in Italian for cranky? Where is this darned place? We almost gave up – particularly when the street numbers didn't match up. But there – at the end of our trek – in plain view for all to see – was Starbene Senza Glutine Panetteria and Pasticceria in all its glory.

If you haven't eaten a cream puff or a croissant in years, then you can understand our excitement to have found this place. The girls picked out several choice items with great glee. We couldn't even wait until we got back to the bus stop, the bus, the parking lot, the car, the highway, the house.... We had to find a café immediately to order tea and coffee so that they could unwrap their treasures and consume them. Needless to say, we made another trip to Florence during the week and made that long walk once again. This time, we also bought some GF ravioli that they had for sale in a cold case in the back. Dinner and dessert in one stop.

Here's an important tip: Gelato is gluten free. You should ask, if you aren't sure, and you should eat your creamy deliciousness out of a cup instead of a cone. Before ordering your favorite flavor, check the beautiful mound of chocolate (or vanilla, or pistachio, or strawberry...) for any errant chunks of cone that might have been accidentally dropped by strong scoopers. Our apartment in Rome had the wonderful Gelato Theatro next door. We tried most of their fabulous flavors. Several times. Per day. All week.

If you wish to travel to far away and exotic destinations, don't give up because of food. Do some internet research and talk to other travelers who have enjoyed whatever locale on your itinerary. Adventures still await you!

Eight

Cooking 101 -

Basic GF Concepts

If you are Julia Childs or Bobby Flay, you can probably skip this chapter.

Gluten free cooking is absolutely no different from any other sort of cooking. You should strive to use the best quality ingredients you can find, the right balance of flavors, along with bold and fearless tastes. Get to know your herbs and spices and don't be afraid to use them. Many of my baked goods that are best sellers in the coffee houses in town (the zucchini toasted almond bread, for example) are selling well to everyone – even people who are able to eat gluten. They like the texture and the flavor. They don't care if it's gluten free or not. This was my goal way back in 2005, when we first landed on this road. I wanted to create foods that everyone can enjoy. So cook away! And you don't have to tell anyone that it's gluten free.

Your kitchen cupboard should have certain essentials. With these you can always put a delicious meal on the table.

- Extra Virgin Olive Oil
- Gluten Free Soy Sauce (San-J Brand is the one we like. Beware of some of the less expensive brands. They are nasty!)
- Kosher Salt
- Black Pepper in a grinder
- Fresh Garlic
- Dijon mustard
- Sriracha (hot chili sauce)
- Dried herbs:
  - Oregano
  - Thyme
  - Rosemary (crushed)
  - Basil
  - Dill
- Spices
  - Cinnamon
  - Ground Cloves
  - Nutmeg
  - Ground Cumin
  - Paprika
  - Chili Powder
  - Ground Ginger (for when you can't manage fresh)

Spices and herbs are expensive, so if you don't have a complete spice rack at this point, add them as you need them. And they don't keep forever, so if the price tag on the bottom of that oregano says, 69¢, you might think about replacing it.

There are usually some dried lentils, canned cannellini and kidney beans, as well as chicken and vegetable stock on our pantry shelves. I love to use homemade stock from bones, but sometimes it's so convenient to have the prepared stock on hand for rice pilaf or a quick pot of soup. Be careful with canned stocks as some of them have gluten. Look for the ones that specify that they are GF.

Fresh herbs have a slightly different impact in a recipe from their dried counterparts (I almost always have fresh parsley, basil, and cilantro in the fridge), but they're not always convenient. Use a 3 times multiplier if you are converting from dried herbs to fresh. Dried herbs will release more of their aromatics if you bruise them in the palm of your hand before adding them to the recipe. Onions, celery, carrots, and bell peppers (green, red, orange, or yellow) are usually in my crisper, along with various greens for salads (spinach, cabbage, romaine, and kale). Frequently some more exotic root vegetables (celery root, parsnips, rutabagas, and turnips) can be found. Added to soups and stews, or just diced and roasted, these ugly guys can really jazz up your meals.

Dinners at our house are sometimes planned well in advance, leaving time to brine the chicken or marinate the lamb chops. But most often, they are last minute creations after work. "Hmm, what do we have in the refrigerator tonight?" Especially when I have been baking all day for the business, I don't really have the energy for coq au vin. From these challenging evenings have come some of my tastiest creations. The trick is to write down what you put into an invented dish while you are making it. Otherwise, it will be a family favorite that you can never duplicate. (Been there. Done that.)

If you have watched any of the cooking shows on TV, you have probably remarked on the incredible knife skills of many of the participants. The speed of the blade blurs. Well, yes, and sometimes the blood flows. But these are important skills that I do not possess. However, learning to cut vegetables (in particular) is still an important part of navigating the kitchen. The rule of thumb that I use is that like items should be similarly sized. First, some cutting definitions.

- Mince – Tiny, like mincing steps.
- Dice – cut the food the size of, well, dice.
- Chop – between dice and cube.
- Rough Chop – Somewhat large, but imperfect pieces – as for sautéed chard.
- Cube – bigger than dice, smaller than a bread box.
- Julienne – long thin strips.

With any completely new dish, it's a good idea to follow the recipe 100%. If you like the first effort, then the second time through might have some adjustments. More or different herbs and spices may be added. Perhaps a different vegetable combination will suit your taste. If it's good with beef, it might also work for tofu, chicken, or pork. The more you work with different ingredients, the more fun you will have inventing wonderful dishes. The heck with gluten!

For the bread loaves, 9X5 loaf pans are the ones indicated in the recipes below. The 9" square pans are for brownies and bars (if you have an 8" square pan, increase the cooking time to accommodate for thicker batter). 8" round cake pans work for the layer cakes. Sheet pans are necessary for cookies as well as confections including caramel, peanut brittle, and toffee. Parchment paper is useful in many different ways. I buy it in 1,000 sheet boxes. A digital food scale is extremely helpful, both for measuring ingredients and for evening out the distribution of cake or bread batter in multiple pans. If you choose to make the toffee, caramel or peanut brittle, you will need a candy thermometer.

Making chicken and broccoli is simple. Baking is a very different animal. Flavors may be changed, but core ingredients must be precise. My lovely Mother was not the best cook (although her beef stew and spaghetti sauce were fabulous), and early in her marriage to my Dad she decided to bake him a birthday cake. She did not have any flour in their little apartment, but since this other ingredient looked somewhat like flour, she figured it would work as well. Baker's Note: Corn starch is not the same thing as flour. She made him a birthday cookie – not a birthday cake. The laughs were worth the effort, apparently.

One of the foremost issues with creating GF baked goods is the texture. It shouldn't be mushy, grainy, overly dense, or heavy. The correct flour blend is important certainly (and you may want to explore making your own flour blend), but leavening is a critical issue. When I was experimenting with some of my old recipes that I wanted to convert, they kept collapsing in the middle. My uneducated answer was to add more leavening. That failed. The correct, counterintuitive response would have been to reduce the amount of baking powder instead of increasing it. Most of the gluten free flours have at least some rice flour in them, and rice flour is not as strong as wheat flour (no gluten, remember?). So, if you add extra teaspoons of baking powder to a rice flour batter, it will create more air bubbles and rise appropriately in the oven, but as it cools, it won't have the internal strength to hold its shape. Fewer teaspoons will still encourage the proper rising and will allow the cake or brownie to sustain its shape. The recipes included later in this book have already had the adjustment made, but if you want to try to make Aunt Muriel's butter cake from her original recipe, you might want to change the amount of leavening.

The blended flours work for many different kinds of cooking projects. As I have mentioned, Tom Sawyer's Gluten Free Flour is my most frequent choice. For pie dough, however, I find that the Namaste Perfect Gluten Free Flour Blend (available at Costco) is better. A few of the recipes that follow ask you to use more than one flour. Sorry about that. Generally, it's the Tom Sawyer's flour and brown rice flour (I use Bob's Red Mill). Only a few recipes (banana walnut bread, for example) use additional xanthan gum. Texture is important.

So, what the heck is xanthan gum, anyway? Can I chew it? Does it come in bubblegum flavor? It appears in so many GF recipes and ingredients. According to Bob's Red Mill's web site (www.bobsredmill.com):

"Xanthan Gum is a plant-based thickening and stabilizing agent. It is named for the bacteria, Xanthomonas campestris, which plays a crucial role in this description. Technically speaking, xanthan gum is a polysaccharide, which is just a fancy way to say "a string of multiple sugars." To create xanthan gum, the Xanthomonas campestris bacterium is allowed to ferment on a sugar. The result is a gel that is then dried and milled to create the powder substance.

Xanthan gum has a number of powerful properties. First, it works as an emulsifier, encouraging liquids that normally don't like one another to mix together. Second, it works as thickener, increasing the viscosity of liquids and batters. Third, it can create a creamy texture.

In the world of gluten-free baking, xanthan gum plays the crucial role of imitating gluten. In baking, gluten is what makes dough "doughy." It gives the dough elasticity, as well as viscosity. Those properties help to hold a cookie together while it bakes on a sheet in the oven, and they enable cakes and breads to hold onto the gas bubbles that form inside them - this allows them to rise and take shape. Xanthan gum helps replicate these properties in recipes that do not contain gluten."

Xanthan gum is expensive. You can buy a small amount. It will keep well in a closed container. It's part of the GF deal.

As you are planning your menu, always review your recipes and verify that you have everything you need. Before you begin to cook, get all of your ingredients out on the counter, along with your pans and measuring equipment. Unless my friend Carlotta lives next door to you, you might not be able to borrow an egg.

So, let's venture forth. Use the recipes that follow and learn how to make everything deliciously gluten free.

Recipes

Oh Good, Now We Get To Cook!

1) Life is short. Let's Make Dessert First
2) Loaves
3) Soups
4) Salads
5) Main Courses
6) Side Dishes
7) Confections
8) Granola – The Beginning and The End

Life is Short -

Let's Make Dessert First

APPLE SPICE CAKE

This cake, when covered with cream cheese frosting is really very special. It has been extremely popular at Wiley's World Restaurant and The Coffee House at Bloomsbury Book Store in Ashland, Oregon for a number of years. In texture, it resembles a carrot cake and it keeps very well when refrigerated or frozen – that is, if it lasts very long!

Ingredients:

2 large eggs
½ cup vegetable oil
1 ¾ cup brown sugar
3 large chopped apples (I use Fuji or honey crisp) – approx. 1 ½ lbs. at the store
1 mashed very ripe banana
1 ½ cup brown rice flour
½ cup Tom Sawyer's Gluten Free Flour
2 tsp. baking soda
1 tsp. salt
2 tsp. cinnamon
2 tsp. vanilla
1 cup chopped walnuts

Method:

Preheat the oven to 350 degrees. Line the bottom of a 10" spring form pan with parchment and spray the sides with cooking spray.

37

Beat the eggs well and add the oil until it is fully incorporated. Add the brown sugar and mix well. Peel the apples, quarter them, and remove the core. Slice each quarter apple thin longitudinally and then again crossways so you end up with little triangles. Add the apples to the batter, followed by the mashed banana. Combine the dry ingredients (flours, soda, salt, and cinnamon) and then fold in to the batter. Finally, stir in the vanilla and the walnuts. Pour the batter into the lined spring form pan and bake for 60-65 minutes. Check doneness with a toothpick. Allow the cake to cool completely, and then remove it from the pan. (Remember to peel off the parchment from the bottom.) You may serve this delightful cake as is, or cover with cream cheese frosting and top with more chopped walnuts. (Note: Because it is very moist, sometimes the cake crumbs pull away with the first coating of frosting which makes the cake look messy, so I allow this to happen and then freeze the cake briefly to set the first coating. Then frost with a second thin layer which covers up the crumbs.)

CREAM CHEESE FROSTING

Ingredients:

6 oz. (1 ½ sticks) softened butter
8 oz. softened cream cheese
1 tsp. vanilla
3 ½ -4 cups powdered sugar

Method:

Allow the butter and cream cheese to come to room temperature so that they are well softened. (You can also help the process along with a few seconds in the microwave.) Cream the butter until it is light and fluffy. Add the cream cheese and beat until it is fully mixed. You don't want to have lumps of butter in the frosting. Add the powdered sugar one cup at a time and then the vanilla. Let the mixer run for several minutes so that your frosting is light and creamy and the sugar is completely melted. Test the texture and add more powdered sugar, if necessary.

This frosting is delicious on the Chunky Apple Spice Cake. It also works well with anything chocolate (layer cake, cupcakes, or brownies).

GRAM'S OLD FASHIONED POUND CAKE

When I was little, we had a very special baby sitter whom we called Gram. She was loving, incredibly fun, and also very strict. I remember her taking my sister and me to the San Francisco Zoo with four other little kids, which would be a daunting task for anyone other than Gram. She always had the most fun outings and we knew that if we misbehaved, we wouldn't be invited again. Gram was also a fabulous baker. Her apple pies were legend. My mother was partial to her buttery pound cake, and Mom could thin-slice a cake to death in very short order. This recipe was derived from Gram's and I think of her every time I make it. For my business, this recipe with the inclusion of lemon has been a best seller. The lemon version follows.

39

Ingredients:

1 pinch of salt
9 large eggs (separated)
¾ cup sugar (for the egg whites)
1 lb. butter (softened)
1 ½ cups sugar (for the butter)
4 cups Tom Sawyer's Gluten Free Flour
1 tsp. gluten free baking powder
1 tsp. vanilla

Method:

Preheat the oven to 325 degrees. Line the bottoms of two 9x5 loaf pans with parchment and grease the sides.

Put the pinch of salt into your stand mixer fixed with the whip attachment. Add the egg whites and beat until frothy. Add ¾ cup sugar to the egg whites and continue beating until they form stiff peaks. Remove the egg white mixture from the mixer into another bowl and set aside. Put the bowl back on the mixer and attach the paddle. (You don't need to wash the bowl at this point.) Put the softened butter into the mixer and beat until creamy. (If your butter isn't pre-softened, you can do so in the microwave for a few seconds.) Add 1 ½ cups of sugar to the butter and beat well. Add 2 cups of the flour to the butter mixture on slow speed (flour can fly all over the place at a higher speed), and then the egg yolks, one at a time. Next, put in the last 2 cups of flour, the baking powder, and the vanilla. The batter will be very thick. Scrape the bottom of the bowl to be sure that all the ingredients are well incorporated. Spoon the reserved egg whites into the mixer and fold in gently at the lowest speed. If you have a 5 qt. mixer, all of the egg whites will not fit into the bowl in one batch and you will have to add the egg whites in stages. Allow the mixer to run for 3 minutes, scraping the bottom several times to be sure that all the ingredients are well combined. Spoon the batter into the prepared loaf pans. (Use your food scale to be sure to have even amounts in the two pans, making sure to tare the scale for each pan.) Bake the cakes for 70-73 minutes, testing for doneness with a toothpick. Allow to cool for 10 minutes before removing the loaves from the pans onto cooling racks. Remove the parchment. Cool the cakes completely before slicing. This cake freezes well, either whole or in portions.

For an alternative, this cake is wonderful with the addition of lemon. Simply add the fine zest (I use a micro plane) of 1 large lemon (approximately 2 Tbls.) and 2 Tbls. of fresh lemon juice (PLEASE don't use that reconstituted stuff. It's terrible.) to the batter above. This cake can also be baked in two 8" round layer cake pans. Reduce the baking time to 45 minutes (test for doneness), and cool completely before frosting.

The lemon pound cake that I sell is frosted with a simple lemon buttercream.

Ingredients:

4 oz. (1 cube) butter (softened)
2 tbls. fine lemon zest
2 tbls. fresh lemon juice
3 ½ -4 cups powdered sugar

Method:

Cream the butter until it's smooth and fluffy. Add the lemon zest and juice and blend well, followed by the powdered sugar. Allow the mixer to run for 3 minutes. Adjust the sugar for the texture that you desire.

CHOCOLATE PASSION CAKE

It's dense. It's rich. It's chocolate. Pure passion.

Ingredients:

8 oz. semi-sweet chocolate chips
1 cup (2 sticks) butter
1 ¼ cups sugar
6 large eggs
1 cup unsweetened cocoa powder
1 tsp. vanilla

Method:

Preheat oven to 375 degrees. Grease the sides of a 10" spring form pan and line the bottom with parchment paper.

Melt the chocolate and butter together (on the stove or in the microwave oven) and blend well. Remove the pan from the heat and add the sugar. Add the eggs one at a time and mix thoroughly. Blend in the cocoa powder (I like to push it through a strainer to remove any lumps). Follow with the vanilla and mix well. Pour the batter into the pan and smooth out to the edges. Bake for 40 minutes. Remove the pan from the oven and allow the cake to cool completely. The cake will collapse slightly as it cools. Remove it from the pan – don't forget to peel off the parchment from the bottom – and transfer the cake to a serving platter. You may enjoy it as-is, dust it with powdered sugar, serve it with vanilla ice cream, or drizzle it with chocolate Ganache (page 46) Another option is to melt some good raspberry preserves in a small sauce pan on the stove and drizzle that over the top. Cut small slices because it's rich, and because that means you will have more left over for breakfast the next day.

CARAMEL PECAN BARS

(Please read this recipe with a Southern accent.) These bars will provide you with the rich flavor of pecan pie in a delightful chewy bar. It's simple to make, and guaranteed to please. All you need is a li'l ole mint julep on the side, and y'all're set to go! Whenever I take these to a food event and provide samples, they always sell out. They're not pretty as a magnolia blossom, but they're yummy.

Ingredients:

 1 cube (4 oz.) butter (softened)
2 cups dark brown sugar
2 large eggs
1 ¼ cup Tom Sawyer's Gluten Free Flour
¼ tsp. salt
1 tsp. baking powder
1 cup chopped pecans
1 tsp. vanilla

Method:

Preheat the oven to 375 degrees. Line a 9" square pan with parchment paper and grease the sides.

Cream the butter until it's light and fluffy. Add the brown sugar and mix well and then the eggs. Combine the dry ingredients (flour, salt, baking powder) and blend into the butter mixture. Add the pecans and vanilla. The batter will be thick. Pour it into the prepared pan, spread it out, and bake for 30-35 minutes. Allow the bars to cool completely in the pan, then remove them and cut them into small squares. You may leave them as they are, or roll them in powdered sugar.

Another dessert option is to bake this batter in a round cake pan, cut the cooled bars into wedges and serve with a scoop of vanilla ice cream and a drizzle of either caramel sauce or chocolate sauce. They are rich and very sweet. A small piece goes a long way.

CHOCOLATE CHIP BLONDIES

Many of my recipes have morphed from one form into another. If you find a combination of ingredients that works, then it's often a good idea to adjust the flavors to create a second version. These blondies are chewy and delicious, and they were the first iteration for the subsequent brownies.

Ingredients:

1 stick (4 oz.) butter
2 cups brown sugar
2 tbls. milk
2 large eggs
½ tsp. salt
1 tsp. baking powder
2 cups Tom Sawyer's Gluten Free Flour
1 tsp. vanilla
1 ¼ cups semi-sweet chocolate chips

Method:

Preheat the oven to 300 degrees. Line a 9" square pan with parchment paper and grease the sides.

Melt the butter in a heavy sauce pan. Add the brown sugar gradually and mix well until the mixture is "gooey". Remove from the heat and add the milk. This will allow the mixture to cool somewhat before adding the eggs one at a time. Pour this mixture into a mixing bowl. You can use your stand mixer or do it by hand. Combine the salt, baking powder, and flour and then add to the butter mixture. Then stir in the vanilla and 1 cup of the chocolate chips. Pour the batter into the pan and sprinkle with the remaining chocolate chips. Bake for 55-60 minutes. Allow to cool in the pan and cut into squares.

BROWNIES

These brownies are rich and fudgy – absolutely great to share. They are delicious as they are or they can have many other alternative flavorings (rocky road, candy cane, triple chocolate).

Ingredients:

1 stick (4 oz.) butter
2 oz. semi-sweet chocolate chips
2 cups brown sugar
2 tbls. milk
2 large eggs
½ tsp. salt
1 tsp. baking powder
¼ tsp. baking soda
1 tsp. vanilla
1 cup Tom Sawyer's Gluten Free flour
1 cup unsweetened cocoa powder
1 cup chopped walnuts

Method:

Preheat oven to 300 degrees. Line a 9" square pan with parchment paper and grease the sides.

Melt the butter and chocolate chips in a heavy sauce pan. Add the brown sugar gradually until the mixture is well incorporated and "gooey". Remove from the heat and mix in the milk. This will allow the mixture to cool sufficiently to add the eggs one at a time. Pour the batter into a mixing bowl (you may use a stand mixer or do it by hand).

Combine the salt, baking powder, soda, cocoa powder, and flour and fold into the chocolate mixture. Then stir in the vanilla and the walnuts. Pour the batter into the pan. Bake for 55-60 minutes. Allow to cool in the pan and cut into squares.

For Rocky Road Brownies: Immediately after baking, sprinkle the top of the hot brownies with mini-marshmallows and bake for another 2-3 minutes. Remove the pan from the oven and allow it to cool completely. Remove the brownies from the pan, dot the top with walnuts, and drizzle with chocolate Ganache (recipe follows).

For Candy Cane Brownies: Omit the walnuts and vanilla from the recipe and replace with 1 cup chocolate chips and 1 tsp. peppermint extract. After baking and cooling, remove the brownies from the pan, drizzle with chocolate Ganache, and top with crushed candy canes.

For Triple Chocolate Brownies: Omit the walnuts from the recipe and replace with 1 cup of chocolate chips (you may use milk chocolate or white chocolate if you like) and top with chocolate Ganache.

CHOCOLATE GANACHE

Ingredients:

4 oz. semi-sweet chocolate chips
3 tbls. butter
1 tbls. milk
1 tbls. honey
½ tsp. vanilla

Method:

Melt the chocolate chips and butter together. Remove from heat and add the milk, honey, and vanilla. Mix well until smooth. Drizzle over cake or brownies, or use as a filling for a layer cake.

CHOCOLATE LAYER CAKE

At the end of World War II, my Dad returned home from his South Pacific service in the Navy. The Navy told all wives to stay put because there was not enough housing in San Francisco for all of them. Mom thought she had a better plan and she left Philadelphia anyway. When she realized that San Francisco had neither snowy winters nor hot, humid summers, she decided that they should stay. Eventually they ended up in an apartment in Park Merced. Their neighbor, Mr. Baade was a creative baker, and he would share his extra cake with the young couple across the hall – as well as his recipes when he had perfected them. This is not his recipe (he requested that none of his creations be shared publicly), but it is a salute to his talent and taste.

Ingredients:

6 oz. (1 ½ sticks) butter, softened
2 ¼ cups sugar
3 large eggs
3 oz. unsweetened baking chocolate
2 cups Tom Sawyer's Gluten Free Flour
1 cup unsweetened cocoa powder
¾ tsp. salt
1 tsp. baking powder
1 ½ cups buttermilk
1 tsp. vanilla
1 tbls. cider vinegar

Method:

Preheat the oven to 375 degrees. Line three 9" cake pans with parchment and grease the sides.

Cream the butter and the sugar until the batter is light and fluffy. Add the eggs one at a time and mix well. Melt the chocolate, (either in the microwave, or very carefully in a sauce pan on the stove. Burnt chocolate does not add to the flavor of this cake.) and stir in the vinegar and the vanilla. Add the chocolate to the butter mixture and mix until fully combined, scraping the bottom and sides of the bowl frequently. Combine the dry ingredients (flour, cocoa powder, salt, and baking powder) and add them alternatively with the buttermilk to the batter. Beat the batter for 3 minutes until it is light and smooth. Pour it into the pans, using your food scale to ensure even distribution. Bake for 30-32 minutes, checking with a toothpick for doneness. Remove the pans from the oven, and allow them to cool for 10 minutes before taking them out of the pans and cooling completely on a rack.

For frosting options, you can use either my Cream Cheese Frosting for filling and topping, or my Chocolate Buttercream Frosting. Alternatively, you can use my Chocolate Ganache for the filling with either of the two frostings.

CHOCOLATE BUTTERCREAM FROSTING

Ingredients:

4 oz. (1 stick) butter, softened
4 oz. semi-sweet chocolate chips
¼ cup heavy cream
½ tsp. vanilla
3 ½ -4 cups powdered sugar

Method:

Cream the butter until it is light. Warm the cream and add the chocolate chips to melt them until they are well combined. Allow the mixture to cool somewhat. Add 2 cups of the powdered sugar (at low speed initially so it doesn't fly all over your kitchen) one cup at a time. Blend the chocolate into the creamed butter and mix well. Add the remaining powdered sugar. (You may adjust the amount of sugar, depending on the thickness of the frosting that you like.) Add the vanilla. Beat the frosting for 3-4 minutes until it is very smooth and fluffy, scraping the bowl frequently.

CHOCOLATE CHIP COOKIES

In college, we called them "Triple Cs" and they were a staple for getting through finals and for impressing the guys in the fraternity up the hill. If you have the patience, and the foresight, it's best to make this dough in advance and let it rest in the refrigerator for at least two hours. Overnight is even better. I use a small ice cream scoop to portion the dough for baking so that the end result is a batch of nice round cookies.

Ingredients:

1 lb. butter, softened
1 ½ cups sugar
1 ½ cups brown sugar
4 large eggs
4 ½ cups Tom Sawyer's Gluten Free Flour
2 tsp. baking soda
1 tsp. salt

4 tsp. vanilla extract
4 cups gluten free crisp brown rice cereal (I use Erewhon brand)
4 cups (24 oz.) semi-sweet chocolate chips

Method:

Cream the butter very well and add the sugars, mixing until the dough is light. Add the eggs and blend well. Combine the flour, soda, and salt and add to the mixing bowl slowly. Beat the dough until it is smooth, scraping the bottom of the bowl to make sure you don't have a glob of butter stuck at the bottom. Add the vanilla. Turn the mixer speed down to low, add the cereal and chocolate chips to the dough, and mix until they are fully combined. Move the dough to a separate bowl, cover with plastic, and chill in the refrigerator for at least 2 hours.

Preheat the oven to 375 degrees (I use the convection setting.). Line the cookie sheets with parchment and portion your dough into the desired size. (A #70 – ½ oz. ice cream scoop makes pop-in-your-mouth sized cookies.) Bake for 8-12 minutes (again, depending on size and chewy or crispy preference) until golden brown. Remove them from the oven and allow them to cool.

One unique option for finishing these cookies is almond toffee. I make the plain toffee (see the Confections section of this book – page 103), and then two minutes before the end of the cooking time, I place a good sized chunk (sized half way between a nickel and a quarter) on top of the cookie. Then finish the baking time. Any more than two minutes will completely melt the toffee and you will lose the special and surprising crunch that it adds. These Toffee Chocolate Chip Cookies sell very well here.

OATMEAL RAISIN COOKIES

These cookies took quite a while to perfect, and the recipe was right under my nose. I had tried to work with an old family recipe that included molasses and lard (don't worry; I never tried it with the lard). They never came out with the right texture. So I finally took my own advice and altered a recipe (the chocolate chip cookies) that already worked, and voila! The flavor of these cookies reminds me of the Dad's Oatmeal Cookies that my father used to buy at the factory in Oakland, California many, many years ago. He had a customer in that area and they sold factory seconds in big brown grocery bags. Delicious.

Ingredients:

1 lb. butter, softened
1 ½ cups sugar
1 ½ cups brown sugar
4 large eggs
4 ½ cups Tom Sawyer's Gluten Free Flour
1 cup gluten free quick oats (Bob's Red Mill)
2 tsp. baking soda
1 tsp. salt
½ tsp. ground cloves
3 tsp. cinnamon
4 tsp. vanilla extract
4 cups raisins
4 cups gluten free crisp brown rice cereal (I use Erewhon brand)

Method:

Cream the butter very well and add the sugars, mixing until the dough is light. Add the eggs and blend well. Combine the flour, oats, soda, spices, and salt and add to the mixing bowl slowly. Beat the dough until it is smooth, scraping the bottom of the bowl to make sure you don't have a glob of butter stuck at the bottom. Add the raisins and the vanilla. Turn the mixer speed down to low, add the cereal to the dough, and mix until it is fully combined. Move the dough to a separate bowl, cover with plastic, and chill in the refrigerator for at least 2 hours (preferably overnight).

Preheat the oven to 375 degrees (I use the convection setting). Line the cookie sheets with parchment and portion your dough into the desired size. (A #70 – ½ oz. ice cream scoop makes pop-in-your-mouth sized cookies.) Bake for 8-12 minutes (again, depending on size) until golden brown. Remove them from the oven and allow them to cool.

CHEWY GINGER COOKIES

These took a few iterations before they were just right, chewy, spicy, and with a crackle top. My Dad loved ginger cookies and I was so glad when they finally came out right. OK, my Dad also loved black walnut cookies, but I'm not going to work on that recipe. I can't stand black walnuts...

Ingredients:

12 oz. (3 sticks) butter, softened
2 cups sugar
½ cup molasses
2 large eggs
5 cups Tom Sawyer's Gluten Free Flour
4 tsp. baking soda
2 tsp. ginger
2 tsp. ground cloves
2 tsp. cinnamon
½ cup large crystal raw sugar (for dipping the dough)

Method:

In your stand mixer, cream the butter well and add the sugar. When that is mixed, add the molasses followed by the eggs. Combine the flour, baking soda, ginger, cinnamon, and cloves together and add to the dough. Blend well. The dough will be firm. Transfer it to a large bowl, cover with plastic wrap, and refrigerate for at least two hours.

Preheat the oven to 375 degrees (I use the convection setting). Line the cookie sheets with parchment and portion your dough into the desired size. (A #70 – ½ oz. ice cream scoop makes a nice sized cookie.) Pour the raw sugar onto a plate and roll the tops of the cookies in the raw sugar. Place them sugar-side-up on the baking sheet. Bake for 8-12 minutes, depending on size and desired texture. If you like a harder ginger snap, then bake them longer. If you like a chewier cookie, then less time is required. Remove them from the oven and allow them to cool.

SPICE CAKE

Spice cake is one of my favorites! It's lovely just plain with powdered sugar sprinkled on top, or a scoop of vanilla ice cream. Cream cheese frosting (see pg. 38) is also a wonderful finish to this moist cake. I also make it with a crumb topping and dust it with powdered sugar and sell it as Spice Coffee Cake. It's a multi-purpose treat.

Ingredients:

2 large eggs
1 cup sugar
½ cup brown sugar

1 cup Tom Sawyer's Gluten Free Flour
2/3 cup brown rice flour
¾ tsp. salt
¼ tsp baking soda
1 tsp. baking powder
½ tsp. ground nutmeg
¼ tsp. ground cloves
1 tsp. cinnamon
1 cup buttermilk
1 tsp. vanilla
2 oz. (half a cube) melted butter

Method:

Preheat the oven to 400 degrees. Line a 9" square baking pan with parchment paper and grease the sides. Set it aside. Beat the eggs with sugars until well combined. In a separate bowl, combine flours, salt, soda, baking powder, nutmeg, cloves and cinnamon. Add the flour mixture to the egg mixture alternatively with the buttermilk, beginning and ending with the dry ingredients. Blend in the vanilla and the melted butter. Pour the batter into the prepared pan and bake for 25-27 minutes. Test the cake for doneness with a toothpick. Allow the cake to cool for 10 minutes and then turn it out onto a rack for complete cooling.

CRUMB TOPPING

Ingredients:

¼ cup brown rice flour
¼ cup brown sugar
¼ cup GF quick oats
¼ tsp. cinnamon
2 tbsp. cold butter

Method:

Preheat the oven to 350 degrees. Put the flour, brown sugar, oats, and cinnamon into your food processor and pulse on and off until it is well blended. Cut the butter into small pieces and process again until it is combined and crumbly. Lightly spray a sheet pan and pour the topping onto the pan. Bake for 15 minutes. Remove the pan from the oven and allow it to cool completely. Crumble half of the topping onto the cake, pressing lightly so that it stays put. (This amount will cover two coffee cakes, so you can use half at once and store the balance in a closed container in the refrigerator.) Sprinkle the top with powdered sugar. I use a sieve and a spoon to get even coverage.

PIE CRUST

This pie crust recipe can be made sweetened (for a dessert pie) or unsweetened (for a quiche). It's simple and delicious. It works well with the Tom Sawyer's Gluten Free Flour, but I discovered that the Namaste Gluten Free Perfect Flour Blend is even better. I know, I wasn't supposed to ask you to buy 27 different kinds of flour…. Sorry.

Ingredients:
1 cup Namaste Gluten Free Perfect Flour Blend
6 tbls. cold butter, cut into small pieces
1 large egg yolk
2 tbls. cold water
Dash of salt
2 tbls. sugar (optional)

Method:

Combine the flour, salt, (sugar), and butter in a medium sized bowl, and blend with an electric mixer until it has a mealy texture. (As an alternative, you can use your food processor). Add the egg yolk and cold water and mix again until it comes together into a ball. Wrap the ball of dough with plastic wrap and place in the refrigerator for at least two hours.

To make a pie, remove the dough from the fridge and let it rest for 30 minutes at room temperature. Roll out the dough between two sheets of plastic wrap until it is approximately ¼ inch thick and appropriately round for your pie pan. The plastic keeps the dough from sticking to your rolling surface and it eliminates the issue of adding more flour through the rolling process. It also makes it easier to fit the dough into the pan. Peel off the top layer of plastic wrap and place the dough into the pie pan. Remove the other sheet of plastic and press the dough into the pan, crimping the edges.

This makes one pie crust. For a two crust pie, double the recipe, form the dough into two balls, and roll out as indicated.

LEMON CUSTARD PIE

Conventional Wisdom indicates that a newly invented recipe should be reserved for a family experiment. It should NEVER be guinea-pigged on a guest. Well then you're not coming to my house for dinner because I do this all the time. Here is one such marvel. It's creamy like cheesecake, lemony and light. Serve it with fresh berries.

Ingredients:

One 9 inch unbaked pie crust (see above)

1/3 cup butter, softened
1 cup sugar
3 large eggs, separated
3 tbls. Tom Sawyer's Gluten Free Flour
¼ tsp. salt
1 tsp. fresh lemon juice
1 tbls. lemon zest
1 ½ cups plain Greek yogurt

Method:

Preheat the oven to 450 degrees. Place the butter into your stand mixer and cream it well. Add the sugar and beat the mixture until it is light. Add the egg yolks and mix until well blended. Add the flour, salt, lemon juice, and lemon zest. Blend in the yogurt. Whip the egg whites until they are stiff and fold them into the batter. (Note: you can add the egg white left over from making the pie crust.)

Pour the batter into the prepared pie crust and bake for 10 minutes. Reduce the oven temperature to 350 degrees and bake for another 45 minutes. The top will be browned. Remove the pie from the oven and allow it to cool completely. The texture is best that way, although we have broken that rule as well.

For all of the recipes that follow, I provide the amounts for two loaves. It doesn't really take any more time to make two, and you can store the second loaf in the refrigerator or the freezer (pre-portioned, if you like), or you can share the second loaf with someone you love.

4/6/16 = Rob VanOrsow Visit
Good- But lots of work

BANANA WALNUT BREAD

Banana bread was the first really good gluten free baked product that I made when we initially ventured into GF Land. It got to the point where my family would stop eating bananas when we got down to three left in the fruit bowl so that they would over ripen – and three was the magic number for making one loaf.

Ingredients:

8 oz. (2 cubes) butter, softened
1 cup sugar
½ cup brown sugar
4 large eggs
2 cups Tom Sawyer's Gluten Free Flour
2 cups brown rice flour
2 tsp. baking soda
1 ½ tsp. xanthan gum
1 tsp. salt
½ cup milk
6 very ripe large bananas, mashed
2 tsp. vanilla
1 cup chopped walnuts

Method:

Preheat the oven to 350 degrees and grease two 9"X5" loaf pans.

In your stand mixer, cream the butter well. Add the sugars and blend until fully incorporated, and then the eggs. In a separate bowl, combine the dry ingredients, flours, baking soda, xanthan gum, and salt. Add half of the dry ingredients to the batter and mix well. Pour in the milk and vanilla. When that is well blended, add the remaining flour mixture. Finally, add the mashed bananas and walnuts. Scrape the bottom of the bowl to make sure that all of the ingredients are mixed well. Then let the mixer run for 2-3 minutes so that the batter is completely combined and there are no chunks of banana. The batter will be thick. Spoon it into the prepared loaf pans and spread the top evenly. (I use a food scale to make certain that the loaves are even. These should be approximately 2 lbs. 8 oz. apiece.) Bake for 62-65 minutes and test for doneness. Allow the bread to cool in the pans for approximately 10 minutes and then turn them out to cool completely.

The texture is best if you let the bread cool, even though it's so tempting to slice into the loaf hot from the oven. Cutting it when it's hot also impacts the moisture and your bread will be dried out tomorrow if you cut in to it too soon today. Patience, my dear, patience.

FRENCH APPLE BREAD

When you find a recipe that works, it's easy to transform it for different flavor options. This is essentially the banana bread recipe that's been morphed into apple. The idea for the ingredients – and therefore the name – came from the little individual pies we used to buy at the corner market after school before we got on the #24 Divisadero bus to go home. Apples, raisins, and spices (especially nutmeg) combine in this moist and flavorful bread. If you really don't like raisins, you can eliminate them.

Ingredients:

8 oz. (2 cubes) butter, softened
1 cup sugar
½ cup brown sugar
4 large eggs
2 cups Tom Sawyer's Gluten Free Flour
2 cups brown rice flour
2 tsp. baking soda
1 ½ tsp. xanthan gum
1 tsp. salt
1 tsp. cinnamon
½ tsp. ground cloves
½ tsp. ground nutmeg
½ cup milk
2 large apples, chopped (I use Fuji or Honey Crisp)
2 cups unsweetened apple sauce
1 cup raisins
2 tsp. vanilla

Method:

Preheat the oven to 350 degrees and grease two 9"X5" loaf pans.

In your stand mixer, cream the butter well. Add the sugars and blend until fully incorporated, and then the eggs. In a separate bowl, combine the dry ingredients, flours, baking soda, xanthan gum, spices, and salt. Add half of the dry ingredients to the batter and mix well. Pour in the milk and vanilla. When that is well blended, add the remaining flour mixture. Finally, add the chopped apples and the raisins. Scrape the bottom of the bowl to make sure that all of the ingredients are mixed well. Then let the mixer run for 2-3 minutes so that the batter is completely combined. The batter will be thick. Spoon it into the prepared loaf pans, and spread the top evenly. (I use a food scale to make certain that the loaves are even. These should be approximately 2 lbs. 8 oz. apiece.) Bake for 62-65 minutes and test for doneness. Allow the bread to cool in the pans for approximately 10 minutes and then turn them out to cool completely.

ZUCCHINI BREAD WITH TOASTED ALMONDS

This bread is enormously popular at the Good Bean Coffee Houses – one in Jacksonville and the other in Medford. Using finely chopped almonds in the batter adds the subtly sweet almond flavor, as opposed to using an overpowering almond extract. Choose organic zucchini if you can. Zucchini is one of the vegetables that is often GMO. This bread is also dairy-free.

Ingredients:

3 large eggs
1 cup vegetable oil
2 cups sugar
3 cups Tom Sawyer's Gluten Free Flour
1 tsp. baking soda
¼ tsp. baking powder
1 tbsp. cinnamon
1 tsp. ground nutmeg
1 tsp. ground cloves
1 tsp. salt
2 cups coarsely grated zucchini
1 ½ cup natural sliced almonds
1 tbsp. vanilla

Method:

Preheat the oven to 350 degrees. Grease two 9"X5" loaf pans. Blend eggs, oil and sugar well. Add the grated zucchini and mix well. In a separate bowl, combine the flour, baking soda, baking powder, spices, and salt. Add the dry ingredients in two portions. Chop 1 cup of the almonds in the food processor and add to the batter. Stir in the vanilla. Pour the batter (which will be fairly loose) into the prepared pans (just a bit less than 2 pounds per loaf – these are smaller loaves than the other sweet breads). Sprinkle the reserved almonds on top. Bake in the preheated oven for 60 minutes. Remove the pans from the oven and allow them to rest for 10 minutes. Take the breads out of the pans and allow them to cool completely before slicing. Do not allow them to cool completely in the pans or they will stick. An alternative to prevent the sticking is lining the bottoms of the pans with parchment.

PUMPKIN BREAD

This used to be a seasonal item for the days when the leaves started to fall, the jack-o-lanterns came out, and the house down the street was decorated with six massive inflated spiders on the roof. But now I bake it year round. Some customers like it with raisins, and some prefer it without.

Ingredients:
¾ cup (1 ½ cubes) butter, softened
1 1/3 cup sugar
1 1/3 cup brown sugar
4 large eggs

3 ½ cups Tom Sawyer's Gluten Free Flour
½ tsp. baking powder
2 tsp. baking soda
2 tsp. salt
2 tsp. cinnamon
1 tsp. ground cloves
1 tsp. ground ginger
2 cups pumpkin puree
1 1/3 cup milk
2 tbsp. brandy
1 cup raisins (optional)

Method:

Preheat the oven to 350 degrees. Grease two 9" X 5" loaf pans.

Combine the flour, baking powder, baking soda, salt, and spices in a large bowl. Set aside. In the stand mixer, cream the butter well and add the sugars, followed by the eggs. Scrape the bottom of the mixer to be sure that all of the ingredients are combined. Add the pumpkin puree. Measure out the milk and add the brandy. Alternating the dry ingredients and the milk, add them to the batter – beginning and ending with dry. If you choose to include the raisins, add them at this point and beat the batter well.

Pour the batter into the greased pans (measure approximately 2 lbs. 8 oz. per loaf) and smooth the tops. Bake for 65 minutes. Test for doneness with a toothpick. Allow the loaves to rest for 10 minutes and then remove them from the pans to cool completely.

CORN BREAD/CORN MUFFINS

With homemade soup or chili, or for breakfast on a Saturday morning, this corn bread is wonderful. You should absolutely break the rule about not cutting into hot bread when it comes out of the oven with this one. A variation with chilies and cheddar cheese follows. I also use this corn bread recipe, plus some herbs, to make garlic herb croutons and, at Thanksgiving, corn bread stuffing mix. Let's just say that the months of October and November are really busy in the kitchen.

Ingredients:

2 large eggs
2 tbsp. sugar
1 cup Tom Sawyer's Gluten Free Flour
2/3 cup corn meal
¾ tsp. salt
¼ tsp. baking soda
2 tsp. baking powder
1 cup buttermilk
½ cup (4 oz.) extra virgin olive oil

Method:

Preheat the oven to 400 degrees. Grease a 9" square baking pan and set aside. (You can also use this for muffins – regular sized or mini.)

Combine the flour, corn meal, salt, baking soda, and baking powder in a bowl and set aside. Beat the eggs and sugar together. Alternating with the buttermilk, add the dry ingredients – beginning and ending with dry. Blend in the olive oil. Pour the batter into whichever pan you have chosen. With muffins, I use an ice cream scoop to more easily portion out the correct amount. Bake the corn bread for 22-25 minutes. Test for doneness with a toothpick. The top should be just starting to turn golden. If you like firmer corn bread let it cook longer.

The muffins take 12-15 minutes. Cut the warm corn bread into squares and serve immediately in a bowl or basket lined with a tea towel. That will keep the bread warmer at the table.

For the croutons, add 1 tsp. each dried basil and garlic powder. Chop ¼ cup fresh parsley (or 1 Tbsp. dried parsley) and add to the batter. Bake the cornbread for 27 or 28 minutes (it will be more cooked and firmer). Allow the cornbread to cool, cut into cubes for croutons, and spread on a parchment paper lined baking sheet. Bake at 250 degrees for a very long time! It will probably take at least 1 ½ hours. Check the croutons periodically and stir them to ensure even baking. They are lovely on soups or salads. For cornbread stuffing, change the herbs to parsley and poultry seasoning. Then when the croutons are toasted, you can use them to make a lovely stuffing for Thanksgiving.

CHILI CHEDDAR CORN MUFFINS

Ingredients:

4 large eggs
3 tbsp. sugar
3 tbsp. diced mild green chilies (canned)
2 cups Tom Sawyer's Gluten Free Flour
1 1/3 cup corn meal
1 tsp. salt
1 tsp. baking soda
4 tsp. baking powder
¾ tsp. red pepper flakes
2 ½ tsp. dried oregano
¾ cup grated sharp cheddar cheese
2 cups buttermilk
½ cup (4 oz.) extra virgin olive oil

Method:

Preheat the oven to 400 degrees. Grease a 24 muffin tin or line with paper liners.

Combine the flour, corn meal, salt, baking soda, baking powder, red pepper flakes, and oregano in a bowl. Mix in the grated cheese and set aside. Beat the eggs and sugar together. Add the chilies to the egg mixture. Alternating with the buttermilk, add the dry ingredients – beginning and ending with dry. Blend in the olive oil. Scoop he batter into the muffin cups. Bake the muffins 12-15 minutes. Test for doneness with a toothpick.

Soups

A big pot of soup is such a welcomed meal on a chilly winter evening. It provides lunch and dinner for the next day as well. Homemade stock is best, but I have used store-bought stock in these recipes.

WINTER CHICKEN SOUP

Cooking with the vegetables of the season will always give you the freshest (and likely, the most locally grown) options. Root vegetables have gotten a bad rap but they can add such a succulent flavor to many dishes.

Ingredients:

4 slices of bacon
½ medium turnip
1 medium celery root
1 medium parsnip
2 medium Yukon gold potatoes
1 red bell pepper
1 medium yellow onion
3 celery stalks
2 quarts chicken stock
1 boneless, skinless chicken breast
2 tsp. dried thyme
2 tsp. dried marjoram
½ cup dry white wine
Salt and pepper to taste

Method:

Cut the bacon into small pieces and place into a large stock pot. While the bacon is frying, peel and dice the turnip, celery root, parsnip, potatoes, bell pepper, onion, and celery stalks. When the bacon is browned, add the diced vegetables and brown them for 3-5 minutes. Dice the chicken breast and add it to the vegetable mixture, stirring until it is no longer pink. Add the wine and herbs and stir well, being sure to scrape the bottom of the pan to release any wonderfulness that has stuck there. Pour in the chicken stock. Stir, cover, and simmer the soup for 30-40 minutes until the vegetables are tender. Check the seasoning and add salt and pepper to taste.

SPICY CHICKEN SOUP

Sriracha is my new best friend. I use it in tuna salad, chicken salad, marinades, and now spicy chicken soup. It adds a little kick (as much or as little as you like) and it has a lovely flavor without all the salt of some other hot sauces. Chicken thighs have a stronger flavor and they hold up to the combination of other ingredients in this soup.

Ingredients:

2 tbls. vegetable oil
4 chicken thighs, boneless and skinless if you can get them
2 large carrots
1 celery root
1 medium yellow onion
2 quarts chicken stock
1- 14 oz. can kidney (or black) beans, drained

1 cup long grain rice (I like Basmati)
2 tsp. dried oregano
1 tsp. cumin
1 tsp. Sriracha hot sauce (or more!)
Salt and pepper to taste

Method:

Cut the chicken thighs into bite sized pieces and set aside. Dice the carrots, celery root, and onion. Heat the vegetable oil in a large soup pot and add the chicken. In 3-4 minutes, add the diced vegetables and brown them for another 3-4 minutes. Add the rice and stir to combine. Pour in the chicken stock and add the oregano, cumin, and Sriracha. Bring the mixture to a boil and then turn down the heat to a simmer. Cook for 15 minutes, until the rice is tender. Add the beans and cook for another 10 minutes.

This soup is lovely served with a dollop of crema (Mexican sour cream) on top and a sprinkling of chopped cilantro. And consider baking a batch of corn bread (see pg. 63) to serve as well.

LENTIL SOUP

Dad used to make lentil soup, usually after we had consumed the Smithfield's ham that Aunt Emmy sent every Christmas. This isn't his recipe, but it makes me think of him whenever the smell fills the house.

Ingredients:

2 tbls. extra virgin olive oil
2 medium carrots
1 medium orange bell pepper
2 cloves fresh garlic, crushed

1 lb. lentils
2 quarts chicken stock
2 cups water
1 tsp. cumin
1 cup cubed ham
Salt and pepper to taste

Method:

Cube the carrots and bell pepper. In a large stock pot, sauté them in the olive oil with the garlic until they are softened. Add the cumin and stir well. Pick through the lentils to ensure that there are no pebbles in the bag and add them along with the stock and the water to the pot. Bring the soup to a boil and then reduce to a simmer, cooking for about 35 minutes, or until the lentils are soft.

Scoop about half of the soup out of the pot and puree it in small amounts in a blender, food processor, or with an immersion blender until it is smooth. Return the pureed lentils back to the pot. Add the ham (or your favorite cooked sausage) to the soup and simmer for another 15 minutes. Add salt and pepper to taste.

If you would like the soup to be a little spicier, you can add a teaspoon of Sriracha, or ½ teaspoon of cayenne pepper.

PHILADELPHIA PEPPER POT SOUP

This was one of Dad's favorites, and once I got past the tripe "ick" factor, one of mine as well. His mother used to make it and he derived this recipe from his memories of her kitchen. The following are his notes from his recipe file:

"It is reliably reported that this recipe was used to feed the near starving Revolutionary War troops at Valley Forge, PA. The British had commandeered all of the choice food while luxuriating in Philadelphia during the winter of 1777-1778. In desperation, the American Troops scrounged every possible source of food and had to settle for anything that remained in the area. The following ingredients were made available by the local farmers having root cellars, preserved vegetables, and organ meats." – Charlie Hoffner

Ingredients:

1 ½ pounds of honeycomb tripe
2 tbls. butter
1 cup tomatoes
2 stalks celery
1 small spicy pepper (we use jalapeno)
1 cup parboiled potatoes (red, or Yukon gold work well)
2 tsp. dried thyme
2 Bay leaves
Salt to taste

Method:

Chop tripe into half inch squares and cover with about 4 cups of lightly salted water in a large pot. Simmer the tripe for 3 hours until tender. Pour the broth and tripe into a large bowl and set aside.

Dice the celery and potatoes. For the tomatoes, peel and seed them before dicing, or you may choose to use canned diced tomatoes instead. Remove the seeds and the veins of the jalapeno pepper and mince. (Note: It's a good idea to wear food prep gloves when you chop any hot pepper. The oil will get on your skin and Heaven help you if you rub your eyes!) Return the pot to the stove and melt the butter. Add the tomatoes, pepper, and celery and sauté them for 2-3 minutes. Pour the tripe and reserved broth, along with the potatoes, thyme and bay leaves into the pot and simmer for 15 minutes. Check the seasoning and adjust the salt to your taste. If you need more liquid, you may add chicken broth so that you don't dilute the flavor.

Salads

Take me out for a meal, even on the coldest winter day, and I'll probably order a salad. We enjoy one nearly every evening with dinner – usually comprised of every vegetable found in the crisper and either a light vinaigrette dressing or a more intense one made with balsamic vinegar and Dijon mustard.

Salads can run the gamut from delicate butter lettuce with sliced avocado and fresh pink grapefruit sections to robust Greek salad with Kalamata olives and feta cheese. Use your imagination, collect the best greens and veggies you can find and go wild. Here are some samples of the salads that frequently grace our table.

FIESTA SLAW

This is wonderful with any Mexican food – part of a basketball team taco bar, served in place of lettuce on tostadas, or underneath a piece of spicy grilled chicken. The recipe is simple, and can be altered to suit your tastes.

Ingredients:

1 large head of cabbage
1 bunch of green onions
1 bunch of fresh cilantro
1 medium jalapeno (or more!)
1 medium red bell pepper
Juice of 3 fresh limes

1 tsp. lime zest
¼ cup extra virgin olive oil
2 tsp. kosher salt
1 tsp. fresh ground black pepper

Method:

Shred the cabbage by cutting it in quarters and removing the core. Slice each quarter thinly and then after it is sliced, once more across in half. Place the cabbage in a very large pot or bowl so that you can stir it easily without spilling out. Chop the green onions, red pepper, and cilantro and add them to the cabbage. After you have seeded and deveined the jalapeno, mince it fine and add it to the pot. The flavor of the jalapeno is essential to the taste of the slaw. Even if you don't care for spicy foods, you must include some of this pepper. Be very careful cutting it, however. Either use food prep gloves, or wash your hands multiple times to remove the oil.

The limes should not be too firm when you choose them or they will not be juicy enough. There should be a little give when you squeeze them. Juice the three limes and add it to the salad along with the olive oil, lime zest, salt and pepper. Mix the slaw thoroughly and then transfer it to a smaller salad bowl for serving. This salad keeps well in the refrigerator, but it must be in an airtight container or it will dry out.

HOFFNER'S FAMOUS COLE SLAW

This is one of Dad's recipes. He always served it with fresh Dungeness crab (cooked, cracked, and eaten in the same day), and a glass of ice cold beer. Now that GF beers on the market are tasting so much better, this meal is a possibility again. It's also delicious with any sort of picnic menu you might put together. This is a wonderful way to use the brine from the dill pickles that you just finished eating. Gourmet Magazine saw fit to publish this recipe in 1981.

Ingredients:

1 large head of cabbage
1 large bunch parsley
3 stalks celery
2 cloves fresh garlic, crushed
1 ½ cups vinegar dressing (recipe follows)
1 ½ cups mayonnaise
1 tbls. celery seed

Method:

Shred the cabbage (see above) thinly and place in a very large bowl. Finely chop the parsley and celery, and add them along with the garlic and celery seed to the cabbage. Pour in the vinegar dressing and mayonnaise and mix well. This slaw really needs a full 24 hours of refrigeration before the flavors marry fully, so transfer it to a smaller bowl, cover tightly with plastic wrap and chill.

DAD'S VINEGAR DRESSING

Ingredients:

1 cup vegetable oil
2 cups white wine vinegar
2/3 cup dill pickle brine (we like Clausen's)
1 tbls. dried oregano
1 tbls. dried basil

½ tsp ground black pepper
1 clove garlic, crushed

Method:

Combine all the ingredients in a quart sized jar and shake well. This makes more dressing than is required for one batch of the slaw. It keeps well in the refrigerator for the next bar-b-que.

*TIP: Another use for your jar of pickle juice after the pickles have been consumed is to slice a yellow onion approximately ¼ inch thick and add the slices to the brine. After two weeks, you will have a jar of delicious pickled onions that are fantastic on sandwiches or as a condiment for any meat.

CHRISTMAS SALAD

This one is a traditional part of our Christmas dinner. It's easy to prepare, festive, and delicious, but not restricted to one particular holiday.

Ingredients:
1 large Romaine lettuce heart
1 ripe but firm pear
½ cup chopped walnuts
¼ cup dried cranberries
¼ cup gorgonzola cheese crumbles (check for GF status)
Vinaigrette dressing

Method:

Wash and dry the lettuce and slice it crossways about 1 inch wide. Add this to your salad bowl along with the walnuts, cranberries, and gorgonzola cheese. Dice the pear and add it to the bowl. Toss with a light vinaigrette (Store bought is OK. You're busy tonight!)

CHUNK SALAD

Although my family enjoys salads, sometimes they are looking for something different. So this one is green salad – hold the lettuce. It's particularly nice in late summer when the tomatoes are really fresh, and genuinely RED.

Ingredients:

2 beefsteak tomatoes
1 large avocado
1 medium red onion
1 green bell pepper
2 stalks celery
1 large carrot
½ of an English cucumber
1 of any other salad vegetable you have in your fridge
¼ cup light vinaigrette dressing
Salt and pepper to taste

Method:

Dice all of the vegetables except the red onion, which should be chopped into smaller pieces. Combine them all in a salad bowl and toss with the dressing.

It's very refreshing and keeps well in the refrigerator for the next day – particularly because my family always picks out all of the avocado.

CARROT MINT SALAD

Many people like carrot raisin salad. Not me. I like carrots and I like raisins – just not together. This alternative combination is light and refreshing and goes well with barbequed ribs or chicken.

Ingredients:
2 large carrots
5 green onions
3 stalks celery
3 tbls. fresh mint leaves
2 tbls. fresh lime juice
1 tbls. rice vinegar
1 tsp. kosher salt
¼ cup vegetable oil
¼ tsp. hot chili oil (Sriracha will work here as well)

Method:
Julienne cut the carrots. (You may cheat here and purchase the pre-shredded carrots at the store. They're not as flavorful and sweet, though.) Chop the green onions, celery, and mint leaves and combine all of the vegetables in a large salad bowl. In a small bowl (or covered jar) combine the lime juice, rice vinegar, vegetable oil, chili oil, and salt. Whisk (or shake) well to combine. Toss the vegetables with the dressing and chill for 30 minutes before serving.

GREEK SALAD

This is lovely by itself, with grilled chicken, or my favorite – with either a lamb burger (see pg. 88) or grilled lamb chop and tzatziki sauce (see pg. 89).

Ingredients:

1 Romaine heart
1 medium tomato
1 small red onion
1 large bunch parsley
1 cup diced English cucumber
10 pitted Kalamata olives
¼ cup crumbled feta cheese
Vinaigrette dressing

Method:

Wash, dry, and slice the Romaine lettuce. Put it in a large salad bowl. Seed and chop the tomato. Finely chop the red onion and the parsley. Add these vegetables to the salad bowl along with the diced cucumber and the crumbled feta cheese. Halve the olives (this will also ensure that there are no accidental pits) and put them into the salad as well. Toss with a light vinaigrette dressing.

QUINOA SALAD

A family favorite, this is essentially a tabouleh salad without the bulgur wheat. When the girls come home from college, it's usually one of their first requests along with "something barbequed".

Ingredients:

1 cup quinoa
2 cups water
1 large bunch of parsley
3 medium tomatoes
1 bunch of green onions
2 tbls. chopped fresh mint
1 cup diced English cucumber
¼ cup extra virgin olive oil
¼ cup fresh lemon juice
1 tsp. lemon zest
1 tsp. kosher salt
1 tsp. fresh ground pepper

Method:

Rinse the quinoa in a sieve thoroughly before it is cooked. Otherwise, it will have a gummy/sticky texture. Bring the water to a boil and add the rinsed quinoa. Bring the mixture back to a boil, reduce the heat, and simmer it covered for 15 minutes.

Chop the parsley, green onions, and fresh mint. Seed and dice the tomatoes. Combine all of these ingredients with the cucumber. After the quinoa has cooked and cooled slightly, toss it into the bowl with the vegetables. Add the olive oil, lemon juice, lemon zest, salt and pepper. Mix well. Chill the salad in the fridge for two hours before serving.

HUMMUS

OK. So it's not really a salad. But it's not dessert or a side dish either. This is such a wonderful dish to make and it has so many uses. This recipe doesn't contain oil, so it's light and fluffy. It's an especially good thing to offer as an hors d'oeuvre with cut vegetables when there are children at the party. If they ruin their appetites for dinner – who cares?

Ingredients:

1 – 15 ½ oz. can of garbanzo beans
2 cloves fresh garlic
2 tbls. fresh lemon juice
2 tbls. sesame tahini
2 tsp. ground cumin
½ tsp. kosher salt
¼ tsp. fresh ground black pepper

Method:

For this, you need to use either an immersion blender or a food processor fitted with the blade. Drain the garbanzo beans, but RESERVE THE JUICE. You really don't want to open another can just for the juice that you poured down the drain, do you?

Put the drained beans, whole cloves of garlic, lemon juice, tahini, salt, pepper, and cumin in the food processor. Pulse on and off until the beans begin to break down. Then turn the machine on and let it run. Add small amounts of the reserved juice from the garbanzo beans to the mixture through the add tube until it reaches the proper consistency (probably 2 tbls.). You can stop the food processor and test the texture and the seasoning. Process it until it's very smooth and creamy. If you like it spicier, you can add more cumin, or some Sriracha.

DRESSINGS

During the week, or when it's a busy kitchen, I often use Girard's Light Champagne Vinaigrette. There. I admitted it. You probably have a bottled dressing that you like too. But it's really very nice when you take a few minutes to create a homemade dressing and immediately pour it on your fresh greens. We have a simple generic dressing that has a few variations.

Ingredients:

¼ cup extra virgin olive oil (gotta use the good stuff!)
2 tbls. vinegar (either balsamic – for a bolder taste, or white wine)
1 tsp. Dijon mustard
1 small clove fresh garlic, crushed
½ tsp. kosher salt
¼ tsp. fresh ground pepper

Method:

Combine all of the ingredients in a small covered jar or plastic container. Shake well and dress the salad immediately. Options for different dressings: Use the lighter white wine vinegar and omit the garlic. The Dijon mustard helps to emulsify the dressing and keeps it from separating. If you like a sweeter flavor, add a teaspoon of honey.

Main Courses

For meat dishes, the simplest and quickest options are usually a simple pork chop or boneless, skinless chicken breast sautéed in extra virgin olive oil, garlic and a few herbs. When the meat is properly cooked, then the pan is deglazed with a splash of white wine. We use the barbeque almost exclusively during the summer and we're charcoal people. It's messy, but so flavorful. We'll have to wait for the second edition of this book for the BBQ recipes!

THE ONE BOWL MEAL

Busy parents can be creative. This one has as many iterations as you have items in your pantry and refrigerator. But it's dinner in a bowl.

Ingredients:

Choose one:

- Roasted diced Potatoes (see pg. 93)
- 2 cups cooked long grain rice
- 1 lb. boiled penne or fusilli pasta

Choose many, diced:

- Celery
- Onion
- Green, yellow, or red bell pepper
- Zucchini or any other squash
- Mushrooms (sliced)

- Eggplant (peeled)
- Carrots
- Any other vegetable in your possession

Choose one:

- Diced, sautéed chicken breast
- Diced ham
- Sliced cooked sausage
- Left-over cooked beef or pork
- Cooked shrimp
- I suppose you could use canned tuna if you like it

Choose one:

- Pesto sauce
- Red pasta sauce in a jar
- Salsa (for a Mexican flair!)
- San-J teriyaki or Thai peanut sauce
- Chopped marinated artichoke hearts with the juice

Choose one (except with the prawns or the San-J Asian sauces):
- ½ cup shredded Parmesan cheese
- ½ cup grated jack or cheddar cheese

Method:

Place the cooked potatoes or rice or pasta in a large mixing bowl. Sauté the diced vegetables in 2 tablespoons extra virgin olive oil until they are tender. Add the vegetables to the bowl. Toss the chosen meat into the sauté pan and warm it also. Add the meat and the selected sauce to the bowl and mix it all well. Test for seasoning and add salt and pepper as needed. Mix in the cheese and you're finished. Dinner!

We also have another version of this dish called Lasasta. You will use the penne pasta and mix in all the other ingredients (pesto or pasta sauce, please). Pour it all into a lightly greased 9X13 pan and cover it with the grated cheese. Bake the dish at 350 degrees for 30-40 minutes.

TACO BAR

Any time the basketball, or soccer, or baseball team is coming over for dinner, a taco bar is always popular and easy. In a group of 15-20 young people, you will probably have two picky eaters and three vegetarians. Set up a taco bar and let the kids build their own dinners to their liking. The quantities below depend on the size of the crowd.

Ingredients:

Taco shells and/or soft corn tortillas
Taco meat (recipe follows)
Shredded lettuce (or Fiesta slaw on page 73)
Grated cheese (cheddar, jack, or cotija cheese)
Canned vegetarian refried beans
Canned pitted black olives
Fresh pico de gallo, or your favorite salsa
Sliced avocado and/or
Guacamole
Sour cream

Put everything out on the kitchen counter with a pile of plates and let the games begin!

TACO MEAT

There are packaged taco seasonings available in the grocery store. Many of them are not gluten free. Why not just use your herbs and spices, plus a little tomato juice and create your own?

Ingredients:

1 lb. lean ground beef or ground turkey or diced chicken breast
1 – 12 oz. can V-8 juice
1 tbls. chili powder
1 tsp. ground cumin
1 tsp. dried oregano

Method:

Brown the meat thoroughly (drain any residual fat). Add the V-8 juice and spices. Bring the mixture to a boil, then turn the heat down to low and simmer for 10-15 minutes until the sauce reduces. I don't usually add Sriracha to this if the gang is coming over. Some people don't like spicy food – and you can always just put the bottle on the table for the adventurous ones in the group.

ENCHILADAS

Make these in advance over the weekend, refrigerate them, and surprise your family on Wednesday night with a delicious fiesta. They are not terribly "saucy", but oh the flavor! You can use almost any filling – cheese, chicken, beef, or pork. This recipe is for chicken.

Ingredients:

1 pkg. of 10 soft corn tortillas
2 boneless, skinless chicken breasts, cubed
½ cup chopped onion
½ cup chopped red bell pepper
1 tbls. vegetable oil
1 tsp. ground cumin
Salt and pepper to taste
¼ cup crema (Mexican sour cream)

Tomatillo Sauce (see below)
½ cup grated cotija cheese

Method:

Sauté the cubed chicken, onion, and red bell pepper in the vegetable oil until fully cooked. Add the cumin, salt and pepper. Transfer the mixture to a bowl and allow it to cool. Stir in the crema.

Prepare the tomatillo sauce and have all of your ingredients on the counter, ready for the assembly line. Lightly spray a 9X13 oven proof dish. Corn tortillas are very brittle, so they need to be softened in order not to break during this process. Place one tortilla in the microwave oven between two paper towels. Nuke it for 10 seconds on high. Remove the tortilla (careful – it's hot) and place another cold one between the paper towels. Warm the second one for 10 seconds while you are filling the first.

Fill the warm tortilla with about ¼ cup of the chicken mixture and roll it up. Place it seam side down in the pan. Repeat with all of the rest of the tortillas. Pour the tomatillo sauce over the tortillas and sprinkle it all with the grated cotija cheese. Cover the pan with foil and bake at 350 degrees for 30 minutes until it is bubbly. Serve with a dollop of the crema.

TOMATILLO SAUCE

Ingredients:

6 tomatillos
1 small jalapeno pepper, seeded and de-veined
1 – 14 oz. can of diced tomatoes, drained
1 clove fresh garlic
1 bunch fresh cilantro
1 tsp. ground coriander

½ tsp. kosher salt
½ tsp. fresh ground black pepper

Method:

Remove the husk from the tomatillos wash and quarter them, cutting out the core. Place them in the food processor fitted with the blade and add all of the other ingredients. Pulse on and off to chop the tomatillos and then allow the food processor to run to make a smooth sauce.

LAMB BURGERS

These are delicious with the Greek salad (see pg. 79) and a tzatziki sauce (which follows).

Ingredients:

1 lb. lean ground lamb
2 tbls. minced shallot
2 tsp. Dijon mustard
2 tbls. chopped parsley
½ tsp. Sriracha (optional)
½ tsp. kosher salt
½ tsp. fresh ground black pepper

Method:

Put all the ingredients in a medium sized mixing bowl. Take off your wedding ring. Put it in your pocket. You really don't want mushed meat on your ring, do you? Mix all of the ingredients with your hands until everything is fully incorporated. Form the meat into three even patties. Or two, if you're really hungry.

Add a drizzle of extra virgin olive oil to a shallow pan and heat it over medium heat until it shimmers. This will get a good caramelization on the meat. Cook the patties in the pan for 3-4 minutes on a side. Touch very gently in the middle to test for doneness.

TZATZIKI SAUCE

When this is served with the lamb burgers and the Greek salad together, it can be a lot of sour things together, so I added honey.

Ingredients:

1 – 6 oz. container of plain Greek yogurt
1 tsp. honey
1 clove fresh garlic, crushed
2 tsp. dried dill
½ cup diced English cucumbers
½ tsp. kosher salt
½ tsp. fresh ground black pepper

Method:

Combine all ingredients in a small bowl and mix well. Either serve it on top of the lamb burger, or in a bowl on the table.

SQUASH CASSEROLE

This tastes better than it sounds. It was even published in Gourmet Magazine (as was the Vegetable Soufflé dish which follows) back in the late 1970s. This dish can be prepared in advance, refrigerated, and baked later.

Ingredients:

1 medium zucchini
1 medium yellow squash
½ lb. fresh white mushrooms
2 medium tomatoes
1 medium onion
1 small green bell pepper
2 stalks celery
1 clove fresh garlic, crushed
1 tbsp. butter
1 cup grated cheddar cheese
1 cup grated Monterey Jack cheese
2 large eggs
2 tbsp. milk
2 tsp. dried basil
2 tsp. dried dill
1 tsp. kosher salt
1 tsp. fresh ground black pepper

Method:

Preheat the oven to 350 degrees. Grease a 9X13 pan and set it aside. Slice the squash, mushrooms, and tomatoes. Mince the onion, celery, and green pepper. Melt the butter and brown the onion, garlic, celery, and green pepper.

Put a layer of the squash on the bottom of the pan (1/2 of the squash), and follow with a layer of the tomatoes and mushrooms. Spoon half of the onion mixture and spread it over the vegetables. Sprinkle half of the cheeses on next. The rest of the sliced squash is the next layer, and then the rest of the onion mixture. Top with the remaining cheese. Beat the eggs, milk, herbs, salt and pepper together and pour over the top of the casserole. Bake the dish uncovered for 30-40 minutes. The vegetables will be slightly al dente.

VEGETABLE SOUFFLE

When your summer garden comes in gang-busters, here's another way to serve that beautiful squash you grew.

Ingredients:

1 large zucchini, sliced thin
2 patty pan squash, sliced thin
¼ lb. white mushrooms, sliced thin
¼ cup finely chopped onion
¼ cup finely chopped green bell pepper
½ cup grated Monterey jack cheese
6 tbls. plus 1 tsp. butter
7 tbls. Tom Sawyer's Gluten Free Flour
1 ½ cup milk
4 large eggs, separated
1 tsp. kosher salt
½ tsp. fresh ground black pepper
¼ tsp. crushed dried Rosemary
¼ tsp. dried basil

Method:

Preheat the oven to 350 degrees. Butter a 5 quart soufflé dish. Melt 6 tablespoons butter over a double boiler and stir in the flour. Slowly pour in the milk and stir until the sauce is smooth and thickened.

Sauté the onion and green pepper in 1 tsp. butter until tender and lightly browned. Add the onion mixture to the white sauce and then the sliced squashes and mushrooms. Fold in the grated cheese and the egg yolks, herbs, salt and pepper. Beat the egg whites with a pinch of salt until they form stiff peaks. Very gently, fold the egg whites into the vegetable mixture. Pour it into the prepared soufflé pan and bake for 50 minutes.

Side Dishes

Side dishes can fill out a more substantial meal, or they often stand very well on their own with a salad for a lighter dinner. You can use these recipes as starting points and build them up with more proteins or vegetables.

OVEN ROASTED POTATOES

We love these. They can also be a part of a One Bowl Meal found in the Main Courses section above.

Ingredients:

2-3 large russet potatoes
1 medium onion (optional)
2 tbsp. extra virgin olive oil
1 tsp. crushed Rosemary
1 tsp. Sriracha (optional)
1 tsp. kosher salt
1 tsp. fresh ground black pepper

Method:

Preheat the oven to 375 degrees. Lightly grease a large baking sheet with vegetable oil or spray. Scrub the potatoes and dice them, leaving the skin on. Dice the onions (if you choose to add them). Toss the potatoes and onions in the olive oil, rosemary, salt and pepper. Pour them onto the baking sheet and cook for 35-40 minutes, turning about half way through, until they are fork tender.

This recipe also works with sweet potatoes (peel them), or any other root vegetables like celery root or parsnips. If you have British friends, they will love you if you roast them some parsnips and Brussels sprouts!

POLENTA WITH MUSHROOMS

Polenta lends itself to many uses. This is one we like very much. If you make a full pot of the polenta, you can save it in a greased loaf pan in the refrigerator for the next morning. Slice the chilled polenta and fry it in a little butter. Delicious by itself or with a fried egg on top.

Ingredients:

1 cup dry polenta
4 cups water
1 tsp. salt
2 tbsp. butter
¼ cup shredded Parmesan cheese

½ pound Crimini or white mushrooms
1 tbsp. extra virgin olive oil
¼ tsp. crushed Rosemary
½ tsp. salt
½ tsp. fresh ground black pepper
¼ cup dry white wine
2 tbsp. sour cream

Method:

Bring the water and 1 tsp. salt to a boil in a double boiler. Slowly add the polenta while stirring. (If you do not have a double boiler, you can use a heavy bottomed pot, but then you must stir the mixture constantly so that it cooks evenly and does not burn.) Cook the polenta for 25-30 minutes until it is thick and creamy. Add the butter and the Parmesan cheese and mix until they are fully melted.

While the polenta is cooking, slice the mushrooms. Sauté them in the olive oil until they become soft. Add the Rosemary, salt and pepper and continue to cook for another 5 minutes. Pour in the wine and allow it to reduce. Just before you are ready to serve the dish, stir in the sour cream.

The mushrooms are delightful served on top of a scoop of the polenta, or some purists prefer to enjoy them separately.

SPOON BREAD

It's bread, with no flour anywhere in the vicinity. It's made with corn meal, milk, and eggs. That means it's really a custard, I suppose. This one is courtesy of Dad and it is light and fluffy.

Ingredients:

1 ½ cups boiling water
1 cup buttermilk
1 cup corn meal
3 large eggs, separated
1 tbsp. melted butter
1 tsp. salt
1 tsp. sugar

1 tsp. baking powder
¼ tsp. baking soda

Method:

Preheat the oven to 375 degrees. Grease a 2 quart casserole. Combine the corn meal and the buttermilk together in a small bowl and mix until there are no lumps. Pour the boiling water into a large bowl and stir the corn meal mixture into the boiling water. Combine the melted butter and the egg yolks. Stir in the salt, sugar, baking powder, and soda into the egg mixture and then add it all to the corn meal. Beat the egg whites until soft peaks form. Gently fold them into the corn meal mixture. Pour the batter into the casserole. Bake for 45-50 minutes.

To quote Dad: "Pretty good stuff!"

WHITE BEANS

Beans are such a great source of protein and fiber. This can be a side dish, a main course as it stands. Ham or sausage can be added if you like.

Ingredients:

1 cup white beans
1 small onion
2 stalks celery
2 medium carrots
1 tbsp. extra virgin olive oil
1 tsp. oregano
½ tsp. kosher salt
½ tsp. fresh ground black pepper
1 qt. vegetable or chicken stock

Method:

Check the beans for any stray pebbles, rinse them and then soak them for 2-3 hours. Dad picked up the trick of boiling twice to remove the (ahem) gas from the beans. So cover the soaked beans in cold water and bring them to a boil for 2-3 minutes in a stock pot. Drain the beans and discard the water. Return the beans to the pot and cover with the stock, bringing them back to a boil. Reduce the heat to low and simmer for one hour.

Chop the onion, celery, and carrots. Sauté them in the olive oil until they have softened. Add the oregano, salt, and pepper and then the vegetable mixture into the beans. Cook it until the beans are tender and most of the liquid has been absorbed.

LENTIL SIDE DISH

Lentils don't take six weeks of soaking (total exaggeration) and ten hours of cooking (another total exaggeration) like beans do, so you can make them without a fortnight's planning before your meal.

Ingredients:

3 medium carrots
1 medium parsnip
1 medium onion
3 stalks of celery
2 tbsp. extra virgin olive oil
2 tbsp. tomato paste
1 cup lentils
1 qt. vegetable broth
1 tsp. curry powder
2 tsp. dried thyme

1 tsp. kosher salt
1 tsp. fresh ground black pepper

Method:

Peel the carrots and parsnip and dice them. Chop the onion and celery. Heat the olive oil to a shimmer in a stock pot and sauté the carrots and parsnips for 3-4 minutes. Add the onion and celery and cook until the vegetables are softening. Add the tomato paste and stir it into the vegetables.

Check the lentils for pebbles, rinse them and add them to the stock pot along with the broth, curry powder, thyme, salt and pepper. Blend the ingredients well and cook on low heat for 35-40 minutes, until the lentils are tender and most of the liquid has been absorbed. Check the seasoning before serving.

Confections

We don't make candy at home, except at Christmas time, and then we place the fudge, caramel, and peanut brittle into charming little festive tins to give away. It's far too tempting to have in the house. We are required to do adequate quality testing prior to gifting, however. The honey vanilla caramel and the almond toffee are regular staples in the commercial kitchen, though. The caramel is very popular at the Rogue Valley Roasting Company coffee house in Ashland, and the toffee is an element of our delightful Toffee Chocolate Chip Cookies.

Candy making isn't difficult, but it can be time consuming and it requires three things – patience, precision, and a good candy thermometer. A gas stove will maintain more even heat than an electric one for any of the temperature sensitive candies. There is something very satisfying about the old fashioned art of candy. The stores are full of packaged confections, but your own are so much tastier. You also have control of your ingredients. There aren't any preservatives in the candies we make. They don't keep forever (if they last that long), but they can be stored in the freezer.

HONEY VANILLA CARAMEL

The version of caramel that is sold at The Rogue Valley Roasting Company (lovingly known as RoCo) is topped with a light sprinkling of Raw Sea Salt. The caramel itself is very sweet, and the coarse grains of salt temper that. It's also fantastic if you drizzle melted semi-sweet chocolate on each piece and top with lightly toasted sliced almonds or half of a pecan.

Ingredients:

¼ cup honey
2/3 cup brown rice syrup (Lundberg Farms)
2 cups sugar
2 cups heavy cream
6 tbls. butter
2 tbls. vanilla

Method:

Line a half sheet pan with aluminum foil and butter the foil. Put the honey, brown rice syrup, and sugar into a heavy sauce pan. Attach the candy thermometer to the side of the pan and place over medium heat. Stir occasionally as the ingredients fully melt and are incorporated into a syrup. Scald the cream over low heat in a small pot. Bring the sugar mixture up to 295 degrees (it will begin to caramelized and turn color as you get close).

Very gradually pour the cream into the sugar mixture. It will bubble and steam like crazy. It's a good idea to have an oven mitt on your stirring hand so it isn't scalded in the process. Eventually it will calm down and begin to thicken. At this point, you need to stir constantly so that the caramel doesn't burn. Bring the temperature back up to 250 degrees (255 if you prefer a firmer caramel). Remove the pot from the heat, take the thermometer out, and stir in the butter and vanilla. Pour the caramel into the prepared sheet pan and spread it evenly to the edges. Allow the candy to cool completely before cutting into bite sized pieces and wrapping the pieces in wax paper or cellophane.

This lovely candy holds up well in the freezer or fridge, but isn't very fond of the heat. So if you make it in August, keep it chilled.

AUNT SOFTER'S FUDGE

I can't explain the name. It's a complicated family story. Just know that Aunt Softer was as lovely as her name sounds and she loved this fudge. It's a very easy recipe – without all the boiling of a traditional cooked recipe. And it comes out perfectly every time.

Ingredients:

8 oz. semi-sweet chocolate chips
4 oz. (1 cube) Butter
10 large marshmallows
2 pasteurized raw eggs, or ½ cup Egg Beaters
1 lb. powdered sugar
1 tsp. vanilla
1 cup chopped walnuts (optional)

Method:

Grease a 9" square pan. Melt the chocolate, butter, and marshmallows over a double boiler. You can do it in a heavy bottomed sauce pan, but it must be over low heat with constant attention. This mixture can burn very easily. After it is melted, remove the pan from the heat and mix in one half of the powdered sugar. In another bowl, stir the other half of the sugar into the eggs/egg substitute. (In the olden days, you could use raw eggs because salmonella was not an issue. You really can't do that now – and you shouldn't. I've had salmonella poisoning and it ain't pretty! As an aside, this is also why I am an evil mother – I never let my children eat raw cookie dough.)

Pour the egg mixture into the chocolate mixture and blend well. Add the vanilla, and the walnuts. It may look a little bit lumpy, but the sugar will melt out into the hot chocolate and become nice and smooth. Pour the fudge into the prepared pan and spread it out to the edges. Allow the fudge to cool completely in the refrigerator covered with plastic wrap. Cut it into small squares and enjoy.

PEANUT BRITTLE

This is the first candy that I made with Dad. And it was a perennial favorite for him and for Mom. We always make it with lots of peanuts.

Ingredients:

1 ½ cup sugar
½ cup corn syrup
½ cup water
2 ½ cups raw Spanish peanuts
1 tsp. salt
2 tbls. butter
1 ½ tsp. baking soda

Method:

Butter two cookie sheets and set them aside. Collect all of your ingredients on the counter before you begin to cook. The process moves quickly as you get to the end.

Put the sugar, corn syrup, and water into a heavy bottomed sauce pan with the candy thermometer in place. Bring the mixture to a boil and cook to 240 degrees. Add the peanuts and salt to the candy and stir continuously up to 300 degrees. Remove the pan from the fire and add the butter, mixing well. Then add the baking soda and combine quickly. It will bubble and get lighter in color (kind of an ugly gray – don't worry, it will settle down when it cools). Pour the brittle onto the cookie sheets and spread it out. Allow the candy to cool and break into pieces. Store it in an air-tight container.

There are brittles made with other nuts and I have tried some. I burned them all. This is a classic, so I stick with it.

ALMOND TOFFEE

This is the toffee that I include in the Toffee Chocolate Chip Cookies (see pg. 49). It's very nice just as it is, broken into irregular pieces, or you can add chocolate and chopped nuts to make a more traditional English toffee.

Ingredients:
2 sticks butter
1 cup sugar
2 tbls. water
½ cup chopped sliced raw almonds

Method:
Grease a large cookie sheet and set aside. Place the butter, sugar and water in a heavy bottomed sauce pan with the candy

thermometer affixed to the side. Stir occasionally as the butter melts and all ingredients are incorporated. Bring the mixture up to 290 degrees without stirring. Add the chopped almonds and stir until just incorporated. The mixture will cool slightly. Bring the temperature up to 300 degrees. Do not stir the candy at this point. If you do, it will separate and your candy will be nasty. When it reaches 300, pour it out onto the cookie sheet and spread it as thin as you would like.

For the chocolate and nut version, immediately sprinkle 2 cups of semi-sweet chocolate chips onto the hot toffee so that they melt. Spread the chocolate out and top with 1 cup of chopped nuts – either more almonds, walnuts, or pecans.

Granola -

The Beginning and the End

This was the first product that I created and it was the first one that was sold to my first customer, the Ashland Food Co-Op. It's wonderfully crunchy and less sweet than more traditional granolas. There is also no added oil or fat – the only fats come from the grains and seeds themselves. I debated whether to include it in this cookbook, because not very many people make their own granola, but it's unique and very popular, so here you go.

GLUTEN FREE GRANOLA

Ingredients:

3 cups Gluten Free Rolled Oats (Bob's Red Mill)
½ cup amaranth
1 cup water
1 cup quinoa flakes
1 cup millet grits
1 cup golden flax seeds
½ cup golden flax meal
1 cup garbanzo bean flour
1 cup brown rice syrup
½ cup maple syrup

Method:

Preheat the oven to 275 degrees. Lightly oil a deep roasting pan and set it aside. Boil the amaranth in the water for 15 minutes until the liquid has been absorbed. In a stand mixer or large mixing bowl, combine the oats, quinoa flakes, millet grits, golden flax seeds, flax meal, and garbanzo bean flour. Add the brown rice syrup, maple syrup, and the boiled amaranth and mix well. Do not over mix or the granola will be too clumpy. Pour the cereal into the prepared pan and bake it for approximately an hour and a half in the following increments:

- 25 minutes
- 20 minutes
- 15 minutes
- 10 minutes
- 10 minutes
- 10 minutes

After each segment, stir the granola well (this is why a baking sheet won't work), making sure to break up any large clumps. Continue baking until the granola is nicely crunchy and turns a toasty golden brown. Allow it to cool completely. It can be stored in a locking plastic bag or a large lidded plastic container. This makes approximately 3 lbs. and it will keep for a long time in the freezer. You do not need to defrost it before eating.

Recipe Index

A.
Almond Toffee, 103
Apple Spice Cake, 37

B.
Banana Walnut Bread, 58
Breads:
      Banana Walnut Bread, 58
      Chili Cheddar Corn Muffins, 65
      Corn Bread, 63
      French Apple Bread, 59
      Pumpkin Bread, 62
      Zucchini Bread, Toasted Almond, 61
Brownies, 45

C.
Cakes:
      Apple Spice Cake, 37
      Chocolate Layer Cake, 47
      Chocolate Passion Cake, 42
      Pound Cake, 39
      Spice Cake, 53
Candies:
      Almond Toffee, 103
      Fudge, 101
      Honey Vanilla Caramel, 99
      Peanut Brittle, 102
Caramel, Honey Vanilla, 99
Caramel Pecan Bars, 43
Chewy Ginger Cookies, 52
Chili Cheddar Corn Muffins, 65
Chocolate Buttercream Frosting, 48
Chocolate Chip Blondies, 44
Chocolate Chip Cookies, 49
Chocolate Ganache, 46

Chocolate Layer Cake, 47
Chocolate Passion Cake, 42
Christmas Salad, 76

Cookies and Bars:
>Brownies, 45
>Caramel Pecan Bars, 43
>Chewy Ginger Cookies, 52
>Chocolate Chip Blondies, 44
>Chocolate Chip Cookies, 49
>Oatmeal Raisin Cookies, 51

Corn Bread, 63
Cream Cheese Frosting, 38

D.
Dad's Vinegar Dressing, 75

E.
Enchiladas, 86

F.
Fiesta Slaw, 73
French Apple Bread, 59
Frostings:
>Chocolate Buttercream, 48
>Chocolate Ganache, 46
>Cream Cheese Frosting, 38

Fudge, 101

G.
Granola, 105
Greek Salad, 79

H.
Hoffner's Famous Slaw, 74
Hummus, 80

L.
Lamb Burgers, 88

Lemon Custard Pie, 56
Lentil Side Dish, 97
Lentil Soup, 69

M.
Main Courses:
      Enchiladas, 86
      Lamb Burgers, 88
      One Bowl Meal, 83
      Squash Casserole, 89
      Taco Bar, 85
      Vegetable Soufflé, 91

O.
Oatmeal Raisin Cookies, 51
One Bowl Meal, 83

P.
Peanut Brittle, 102
Philadelphia Pepper Pot Soup, 70
Pie Crust, 55
Polenta with Mushrooms, 94
Potatoes, Oven Roasted, 93
Pumpkin Bread, 62

Q.
Quinoa Salad, 79

S.
Salad Dressings, 82
Salads:
      Carrot Mint Salad, 78
      Christmas Salad, 76
      Chunk Salad, 77
      Dad's Vinegar Dressing, 75
      Fiesta Slaw, 73
      Greek Salad, 79
      Hoffner's Famous Slaw, 74
      Quinoa Salad, 79

Side Dishes:

       Lentil Side Dish, 97
       Polenta with Mushrooms, 94
       Potatoes, Oven Roasted, 93
       Spoon Bread, 95
       White Bean Side Dish, 96

Soups:

       Lentil Soup, 69
       Philadelphia Pepper Pot Soup, 70
       Spicy Chicken Soup, 68
       Winter Chicken Soup, 67

Spice Cake, 53
Spicy Chicken Soup, 68
Spoon Bread, 95
Squash Casserole, 89

T.

Taco Bar, 85
Tomatillo Sauce, 87
Tzatziki Sauce, 89

V.

Vegetable Soufflé, 91

W.

White Bean Side Dish, 96
Winter Chicken Soup, 67

Z.

Zucchini Bread, Toasted Almond, 61

Gluten Free Guide
AND
Cook Book

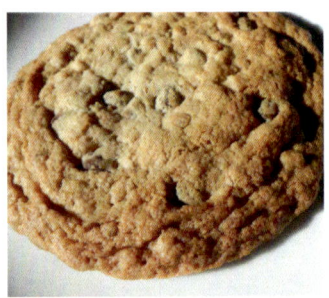

Nancy Shulenberger is the owner of the *Sterling Silver Food Company* based in the beautiful Rogue Valley in Southern Oregon. She grew up in San Francisco, earned a BA from the University of California at Berkeley, and lived, cooked, and dined most of her adult life in the San Francisco Bay Area. Nancy's two daughters were diagnosed with Celiac Disease in middle school. Four years later, the Shulenberger family moved to Ashland, Oregon where the Sterling Silver Food Company was born.

From granola to the mighty chocolate chip cookie, the Sterling Silver Food Company produces much-loved gluten free products. Since the company's inception in 2010, nearly a ton of granola and more than 33,000 individual baked goods have made a difference in our customers' lives. We can help you too.

This is a perfect gift for the gluten free community!

Are you overwhelmed by a diagnosis of Celiac Disease or gluten intolerance?

Can you manage a gluten free diet?

Will you ever eat again?

Do you have concerns about any of these?
- Dining Out
- Travel
- GF & Kids

This book provides you with a simple and comprehensive understanding of a deliciously gluten free existence in a gluten full world.

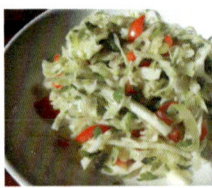

$14.95
ISBN 978-0-9904234-0-9

9 780990 423409

51495>

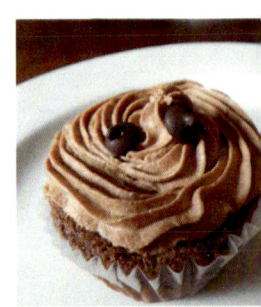